LOWER EXTREMITY TRAUMA

LOWER EXTREMITY TRAUMA

Edited by

Milton B. Armstrong
University of Miami
Miami, Florida, U.S.A.

informa
healthcare

New York London

Informa Healthcare USA, Inc.
270 Madison Avenue
New York, NY 10016

Printed in the United States of America on acid-free paper
10 9 8 7 6 5 4 3 2 1

International Standard Book Number-10: 0-8247-2865-3 (Hardcover)
International Standard Book Number-13: 978-0-8247-2865-6 (Hardcover)

Visit the Informa Web site at
www.informa.com

and the Informa Healthcare Web site at
www.informahealthcare.com

To my sons Christopher and Bryan;
to my parents, James and Cornelia Armstrong, for their guidance, love, and support;
to Annette, Jauqua, and Khara for all of their love;
to my immediate family, for their encouragement of all my efforts.

Preface

Increasingly, urban trauma is becoming a major health care issue. Large emergency departments are inundated with patients with multiple injuries, requiring state-of-the-art care. Most of these complex injuries involve trauma to the extremities, often due to motor vehicle accidents. In a study by MacKenzie et al. (1), it was shown that lower extremity injuries accounted for about 40% of the charges for motor vehicle trauma treatment in a given year.

This book is designed to be a guide for the evaluation and management by physicians, nurses, students, and support personnel involved in the care of severely injured patients. I am very pleased to have an outstanding group of contributors from the University of Miami/Jackson Memorial Hospital Medical Center. University of Miami/Jackson Memorial Hospital serves as the primary Level 1 trauma referral center for South Florida. With such a tremendous volume of trauma patients, University of Miami/Jackson Memorial Hospital and its staff manages some of the most complicated lower extremity trauma problems on a daily basis.

University of Miami/Jackson Memorial Hospital employs a comprehensive system that allows for the coordination of care amongst multiple surgical services. These services include trauma/critical care, orthopedic trauma, vascular, and plastic surgery—all areas thoroughly covered within this text.

Milton B. Armstrong

REFERENCE

1. MacKenzie EJ, Cushing BM, Jurkovich GJ, et al. Physical impairment and functional outcomes six months after severe lower extremity fractures. J Trauma 1993; 34(4): 528–539.

Acknowledgments

I am deeply indebted to my current and former University of Miami residents and fellows, my colleagues in the University of Miami Division of Plastic Surgery, the University of Miami Department of Surgery, and contributing authors from around the country.

Contents

Contributors

Milton B. Armstrong Division of Plastic Surgery, Miller School of Medicine, University of Miami, Miami, Florida, U.S.A.

Efrain Arias Florida State University College of Medicine, Tallahassee, Florida, U.S.A.

Malachy E. Asuku Department of Plastic and Reconstructive Surgery, Ahmadu Bello University Teaching Hospital, Kaduna, Nigeria

Marcelo Lacayo Baez Universidad Autonoma de Guadalajara, Guadalajara, Mexico

Mark Cockburn Department of Surgery, Morristown Memorial Hospital, Morristown, New Jersey, U.S.A.

Stephen M. Cohn Divisions of Trauma and Surgical Critical Care, Miller School of Medicine, University of Miami, Miami, Florida, U.S.A.

Darwin Eton Miller School of Medicine, University of Miami, Miami, Florida, U.S.A.

Jonathan Fisher Division of Plastic Surgery, Miller School of Medicine, University of Miami, Miami, Florida, U.S.A.

Fahim A. Habib Division of Trauma and Surgical Critical Care, DeWitt Daughtry Department of Surgery, Miller School of Medicine, University of Miami, Miami, Florida, U.S.A.

Igor Jeroukhimov Divisions of Trauma and Surgical Critical Care, Miller School of Medicine, University of Miami, Miami, Florida, U.S.A.

Steven P. Kalandiak Department of Orthopedics and Rehabilitation, Miller School of Medicine, University of Miami, Miami, Florida, U.S.A.

Yoram Klein Divisions of Trauma and Surgical Critical Care, Miller School of Medicine, University of Miami, Miami, Florida, U.S.A.

Joshua Kreithen Division of Plastic Surgery, University of Florida School of Medicine, Gainesville, Florida, U.S.A.

Sabrina Lahiri Division of Plastic Surgery, Miller School of Medicine, University of Miami, Miami, Florida, U.S.A.

Kerry Latham Division of Plastic Surgery, Miller School of Medicine, University of Miami, Miami, Florida, U.S.A.

Robert L. McCauley Department of Plastic and Reconstructive Surgery, Shriners Burns Hospital, Surgery and Pediatrics, University of Texas Medical Branch, Galveston, Texas, U.S.A.

Seung-Jun O Division of Plastic Surgery, Medical University of South Carolina, Charleston, South Carolina, U.S.A.

Anire Okpaku Department of Surgery, Jackson Memorial Hospital, Miller School of Medicine, University of Miami, Miami, Florida, U.S.A.

Zubin J. Panthaki Departments of Clinical Surgery, Clinical Orthopedics, and Rehabilitation, Division of Plastic and Hand Surgery, DeWitt Daughtry Family Department of Surgery, Miller School of Medicine, University of Miami, Miami, Florida, U.S.A.

Pranay Ramdev Division of Vascular Surgery, DeWitt Daughtry Department of Surgery, Miller School of Medicine, University of Miami, Miami, Florida, U.S.A.

Rajeev Venugopal Department of Surgery, University of the West Indies, Jamaica, West Indies

Kerri Woodberry Division of Plastic Surgery, Saint Louis University School of Medicine, St. Louis, Missouri, U.S.A.

1

Basic Principles of Trauma Care

Yoram Klein, Igor Jeroukhimov, and Stephen M. Cohn

Divisions of Trauma and Surgical Critical Care, Miller School of Medicine, University of Miami, Miami, Florida, U.S.A.

Mark Cockburn

Department of Surgery, Morristown Memorial Hospital, Morristown, New Jersey, U.S.A.

OVERVIEW

In the United States, trauma constitutes the third major cause of death of all ages and the leading cause of death among persons less than 44 years old (1). Currently, more than 400 people die of injuries in the United States every day (2) and about 50% of these deaths occur prior to hospital arrival. The major causes of trauma-related death are devastating injury of the central nervous system (CNS) (50%) and uncontrolled hemorrhage (35%) (3). Thirty-seven million people are treated for injuries in emergency departments each year, accounting for 37% of all emergency department visits of which 2.6 million require hospitalization. The total cost associated with injuries is estimated to be more than $250 billion per year.

Satisfactory outcomes for injured patients are strongly influenced by the initial care delivered following admission to the hospital emergency department (4). Approximately 60% of all trauma-related hospital deaths occur during the first hour. Inadequate assessment and resuscitation contributes to a preventable death rate of about 35% (5).

A schematic approach for the treatment of severely injured patients consists of triage, primary survey, resuscitation, secondary survey, monitoring and evaluation, and transfer to definitive care (6).

The primary survey is performed to identify immediately the life-threatening injuries:

1. Airway control with cervical spine protection,
2. Breathing and ventilation,
3. Circulation with hemorrhage control,
4. Disability: neurologic status, and
5. Exposure/environment control.

The primary survey and resuscitation are performed simultaneously. The secondary survey consists of obtaining a complete history and a "head-to-toe" examination following the primary survey. Frequent reevaluation is performed to recognize and treat any deterioration in the patient's condition.

The modern concept of initial trauma care focuses on the physiological derangements following severe trauma, rather than the specific injuries sustained by the patient. A thorough understanding of the basic management principles of the multi-injured trauma patient is therefore essential for successful treatment of the patient with severe lower extremity trauma. In contrast, certain lower extremity injuries are specifically associated with dangerous systemic effects. Every physician who takes care of trauma patients should be acquainted with these injuries and their management.

AIRWAY MANAGEMENT IN THE TRAUMA SETTING

The first priority in the treatment of trauma patients is to establish airway patency, because obstructed upper airway will cause almost immediate hypoxia and respiratory acidosis. Posterior displacement of the tongue due to loss of muscle tone in comatose patients, and obstructive particles such as tissue debris, vomitus, or foreign bodies are the most common causes for upper airway obstruction in trauma patients.

Cervical spine injuries occur in 1.5% to 3% of blunt trauma victims, of which 25% to 75% are unstable (7–9). Patients with clinically significant head trauma may have a greater risk of cervical spine injury (4.9% vs. 1.1% without head injury), and the incidence increases to 7.8% in trauma victims with a Glasgow coma score (GCS) less than 8 (10). These facts make the presence of unstable cervical spine fracture relatively common in trauma patients that require airway control. Until cervical spine instability is ruled out, neck immobilization should be maintained at all times. During airway management, neck manipulation is common. Minimizing unnecessary neck movement is best achieved with a minimum of two persons, because one of them is committed exclusively to maintaining in-line neck immobilization (11).

Overt signs of airway obstruction may be complete with apnea, marked cyanosis, or stridor. More subtle signs such as labored ventilation, hoarseness, or use of accessory muscles of ventilation may suggest incomplete or milder airway obstruction. Finally, severe oromaxillofacial injury or burn are situations associated with pending airway obstruction, and securing the airway in these circumstances should be performed prior to clinical signs of obstruction.

After evacuating the airway of foreign bodies, tissue debris, or vomited material, a jaw thrust or chin lift maneuver, followed by the insertion of a short oropharyngeal airway tube may quickly alleviate obstruction due to tissue laxity or posterior displacement of the tongue. These techniques are temporary airway control maneuvers. If airway obstruction is not resolved using this simple technique, definitive airway control should be achieved promptly by endotracheal intubation or a surgical airway procedure.

Indications for Intubation

Intubation is reserved for those patients who continue to show signs of inadequate respiration after basic interventions or those in whom these interventions alone are not likely to sustain appropriate respiration (12).

Absolute Indications for Intubation:

1. Airway obstruction unrelieved with basic interventions,
2. Apnea or near apnea,
3. Respiratory distress, and
4. Severe neurologic deficit or decreased consciousness (i.e., focal deficit or GCS rating less than 9) due to head trauma or any other cause.

Urgent Indications for Intubation:

1. Penetrating neck injury (with any signs of airway compromise or expanding hematoma),
2. Persistent or refractory hypotension, especially due to active hemorrhage,
3. Chest wall injury with respiratory dysfunction, and
4. Moderate altered mentation, especially after head trauma, including both combative and mildly obtunded patients.

Relative Indications for Nonemergent Intubation:

1. Oromaxillofacial injury,
2. Impending respiratory failure,
3. Need for diagnostic or therapeutic procedures [e.g., computed tomography (CT) or angiography] in patients with risk for deterioration or those unable to remain motionless during the examination, and
4. Potential respiratory failure after sedative-analgesic use.

Direct Orotracheal Intubation

All victims of blunt trauma undergoing urgent intubation should be regarded as having a cervical spine injury until proven otherwise. Preoxygenation should be performed in trauma patients prior to intubation. Oral endotracheal intubation with manual in-line stabilization of the cervical spine is the most rapid and reliable method to secure the airway of the apneic patient. This approach is superior to blind nasal intubation in terms of safety, success rate, time to intubation, and number of attempts required. In the optimal situation, three people are necessary to perform a successful intubation: (i) to perform laryngoscopy and intubation, (ii) to provide cervical spine immobilization, and (iii) to apply cricoid pressure (picture). Suction devices should be readily available prior to an attempt at intubation whenever possible. Pharmacological agents that include short-acting muscle relaxants and sedatives may be given as part of the rapid sequence intubation, which is considered to be the proper approach for urgent intubation in the trauma setup (13).

Nasal Intubation

Nasal intubation has no advantages over oral intubation, may be technically more difficult, and should not be performed in trauma patients. Nasal intubation is performed in a "blind" fashion, can only be performed in spontaneously breathing patients, and should not be used in the presence of face, head, and neck injuries. The success rate for this procedure is significantly lower (65%), and requires more time than for orotracheal intubation (14). Two cases of death from airway obstruction after nasal intubation have been reported (15).

Laryngeal Mask Airway

A laryngeal mask airway (LMA) device may be inserted with the head secured in neutral position without using muscle relaxants (16,17). Experience with LMA in elective anesthesia revealed a few benefits that make the LMA an appealing alternative to endotracheal intubation in trauma care, especially in the prehospital setting. These benefits include airway and cervical muscle tone preservation, avoidance of right main stem bronchus intubation, and low incidence of aspiration (18). However, no study has demonstrated that a properly placed LMA provides better airway protection than oral airway and bag/mask ventilation in the setting of trauma.

Surgical Airway

A surgical airway is necessary when basic interventions and intubation are not successful (e.g., in cases of severe anatomic distortion of the upper airway from middle or lower facial trauma) (12). At our center with excellent anesthesiology support services, we rarely have needed to perform a surgical airway (0.3% of trauma intubations).

Cricothyroidotomy

Cricothyroidotomy is the surgical airway of choice because it is simple, easy to perform, and relatively safe in the trauma setting. One must first identify anatomic landmarks (i.e., palpation of the thyroid cartilage and cricothyroid membrane). A vertical incision is then made from the thyroid cartilage to the cricoid cartilage. The cricothyroid membrane is identified and a 1.5- to 2-cm transverse incision is made through the membrane followed by introduction of an endotracheal tube (usually size 6 mm) into the airway. The complication rate of cricothyroidotomy in the trauma setting approaches 39% (15) and includes minor hemorrhage, hypoxia secondary to prolonged procedure time, misplacement, esophageal perforation, laryngeal fracture, thyroid bleeding, and emphysema. Care must be taken to avoid lateral dissection and low incision. There are anecdotal reports that subglottic stenosis may develop after cricothyroidotomy. This has been postulated to result from prolonged insertion time resulting in ischemia or error in surgical technique. Because of the smaller size and greater soft tissue compliance of the pediatric airway, as well as the greater importance of the cricoid cartilage in maintaining patency of the tracheal lumen, this procedure is relatively contraindicated in pediatric trauma patients. Particularly in children 12 years old or younger, needle cricothyroidotomy with later conversion to tracheostomy is utilized to avoid subglottic stenosis (19).

Percutaneous Translaryngeal Catheter Insufflation

A large-bore (12–14 guage) needle may be inserted into the relatively avascular cricothyroid membrane, which is located between the shield-shaped thyroid cartilage and the interiorly located ring-shaped cricoid cartilage. This can serve as a temporary measure to oxygenate a patient prior to establishing a definitive airway.

High-pressure or jet insufflation may lead to horrific complications (subcutaneous emphysema, pneumathorax, pneumomediastinum, and neck hematoma from injured thyroid vessels) and should never be used in the trauma setting.

Tracheostomy

Tracheostomy is a poor choice of procedure for emergent airway control. The trachea lies deep in the neck surrounded by an extensive vascular supply and the isthmus of thyroid gland. Tracheostomy may be required in patients with acute laryngeal trauma in whom placement of a tube through the cricothyroid may complicate existing laryngeal injury.

BREATHING AND VENTILATION

Four major pathologic conditions affecting the respiratory system should be recognized during the primary trauma assessment: tension pneumothorax, open pneumothorax, massive hemothorax, and flail chest. Tension pneumothorax is a clinical diagnosis characterized by chest pain, signs of respiratory compromise, tachycardia, hypotension, absence of unilateral breath sounds, and later, tracheal deviation and neck vein distention. Treatment consists of immediate large-bore needle decompression of the pleural cavity in the second intercostal space, midclavicular line followed by chest tube insertion. Open pneumothorax results from a traumatic defect of the chest wall large enough to permit air to enter into the pleural cavity. If the opening in the chest wall exceeds two-thirds the diameter of the trachea, air passes preferentially through the chest defect with every respiratory effort, creating the so-called "sucking chest wound." Initial management includes prompt occlusion of the wound with a large dressing, overlapping the wound's edges, and taped securely on three sides to provide a flutter-type valve effect. A chest tube should be placed immediately in order to prevent rapid development of a tension pneumothorax. The chest tube should be inserted remote from the wound. In patients with a flail chest injury, an unstable segment of the normally rigid chest wall moves "paradoxically," in an opposite direction from the rest of the thoracic cage during the respiratory cycle. While a relatively unusual injury seen in only 5% to 13% of the patients with chest trauma (20,21), flail chest is a marker for other significant injuries, specifically underlying lung contusion. Pulmonary contusion accompanies about one-half of flail chest injuries and is the major cause of hypoxia in these patients. Diagnosis of flail chest is based on clinical findings of a paradoxically moving segment of the chest wall accompanied by rib crepitus and local pain, and is confirmed with chest X ray. More than 70% of patients with flail chest have a pneumothorax and/or hemothorax (22,23). Massive hemothorax results from the rapid accumulation of more than 1500 mL of blood in the pleural cavity. Clinically, massive hemothorax is usually associated with symptoms of hypovolemic shock, absent breath sounds, and dullness to percussion over the lesion. Treatment consists of simultaneous decompression of the involved pleural cavity and restoration of circulating blood volume.

The most common device used for supporting ventilation is the bag-valve mask device (BVM). BVM ventilation is extremely effective but requires careful attention to maintain a tight mask seal, airway patency, and delivery of adequate tidal volume. The BVM device should be attached to high-flow supplemental oxygen with delivery of at least 15 L/min to avoid hypoxia. Even in skilled hands, BVM ventilation requires continuous monitoring of mask seal, airway patency, tidal volume, the presence of foreign material, and gastric insufflation. In patients with severe midface injury, a mask seal may be difficult to maintain. If adequate ventilation is unsuccessful with the BVM device, immediate intubation or surgical airway should be performed.

ASSESSMENT OF CIRCULATORY STATUS AND HEMORRHAGE CONTROL

After proper airway control and respiratory management, initial assessment of the circulatory status is required. The initial diagnosis of shock (inadequate delivery of oxygen to the tissues) is based on clinical signs not laboratory data. Signs of hypoperfusion should lead to immediate initiation of resuscitation and investigation into the source of blood loss. Hemorrhage and hypovolemia are by far the most common etiology for shock in the trauma setting. Rarely these patients may present to the hospital after trauma with neurogenic, cardiogenic, or even septic shock. Organ hypoperfusion does not result from isolated brain injury but can result from spinal cord injury, resulting in the loss of sympathetic tone. Cardiogenic shock may rarely result from direct myocardial injury, but more likely from an acute ischemic event secondary to hypovolemia or hypoxemia. Septic shock is very unusual except in patients whose arrival has been delayed for many hours or days.

Hemorrhage is therefore the most common cause of shock in trauma patients. Thirty-five percent of all trauma-related deaths in the prehospital setting occur from uncontrolled hemorrhage. Profound hemorrhagic shock can be easily recognized because of obvious signs of inadequate perfusion of the CNS and skin. Hypotension is not manifested until more than 25% of the blood volume (20 cm^3/kg BW or 1500 cm^3 in a 70-kg patient) is lost. Therefore, subtle signs of occult hemorrhage such as agitation and mild increase in heart rate should be recognized as possible early signs of blood loss. Base deficit should be assessed by arterial blood gas (ABG) analysis upon arrival and serially to aid in the diagnosis of metabolic acidosis secondary to hypovolemia. Two large-bore venous catheters should be placed to achieve optimal access for fluid resuscitation.

The patient's response to initial fluid resuscitation is the key determinant guiding further therapy. A rough guideline of the total amount required for crystalloid resuscitation is to replace every milliliter of blood lost with 3 mL of crystalloid fluid, thus allowing replenishment of plasma volume and accounting for fluid loss to the interstitial and intracellular spaces. The decision to start the infusion of blood is based on the patient's failure to respond to the initial fluid bolus. The primary purpose of blood administration is to provide additional oxygen-carrying capacity and to restore circulating volume. Fully cross-matched blood is preferred, but cross-matching requires 45 minutes to complete. Type-specific blood can be provided within 10 minutes and this blood is compatible with ABO and Rh blood types. When type-specific blood is unavailable, type O packed red blood cells are utilized for unstable patients with life-threatening hemorrhage. Thus, the initial management goals in the care of the trauma victim with hemorrhagic shock include resuscitation, identification of the source of bleeding, and achieving hemostasis. Significant hemorrhage in a trauma patient may occur at multiple locations including external bleeding; intracavitary hemorrhage into the pleural space or peritoneal cavity; bleeding into muscle and subcutaneous tissue from contusions and fractures; and bleeding into the retroperitoneum.

External hemorrhage from wounds is usually obvious and can be controlled by direct pressure. There are rare situations in which a tourniquet should be applied proximal to the site of bleeding to control blood loss while other life-threatening conditions are addressed, during the triage phase of mass casualties or in hostile environments. A tourniquet produces distal ischemia (which will become irreversible within six to eight hours), increases local tissue damage, and should be the last resort used only in extreme situations as mentioned above.

Bleeding into the pleural cavity from the mediastinal large vessels like the aorta or pulmonary vessels is universally fatal. Bleeding from smaller vessels (intercostals or internal mammary) or from the lung's parenchyma can produce a hemothorax, which can be easily diagnosed by clinical examination and chest X ray. Less than 10% of patients with traumatic hemothorax require thoracotomy. The remainder can be treated by thoracostomy tube drainage alone.

Substantial intra-abdominal blood loss can occur without obvious clinical signs. Hemoperitoneum may be easily diagnosed by abdominal ultrasonography or diagnostic peritoneal lavage. Only stable patients are able to undergo abdominal CT. Patients in shock with hemoperitoneum require urgent laparotomy.

The retroperitoneum is another important source of bleeding in abdominal trauma. The most common causes of retroperitoneal hemorrhage are the pelvis, the kidneys, and small vessels in the iliopsoas region. Due to the retroperitoneal confined space, bleeding events are most commonly self-limiting, and exploration and surgical hemostasis are rarely required.

Pelvic fracture with massive bleeding is a complicated and life-threatening situation. Although more than 90% of cases of bleeding from pelvic fracture are of venous origin, arterial bleeding may cause severe hemorrhagic shock. The method of choice for bleeding control is angiographic embolization, while other methods such as anterior external fixation, C-clamp, application of pelvic binder, or pneumatic antishock garment are controversial adjuncts to the initial management of these patients (24).

Reassessment of the adequacy of resuscitation is essential to prevent organ dysfunction. Persistence of significant base deficits, uncorrectable lactic acidosis, and oliguria are all indicators of inadequate resuscitation. The initial goal in volume resuscitation should be restoration of organ perfusion rather than increased blood pressure. Serial examinations should be performed to identify evidence of ongoing hemorrhage, such as hypothermia, coagulopathy, and metabolic acidosis. Patients must be maintained in a warm environment and infused solutions heated to 39°C before administration. Transfusion of coagulation factors, fresh-frozen plasma, and platelets is guided by clinical coagulation status supplemented by laboratory tests. Certainly, all efforts should be directed toward controlling hemorrhage rather than treating its complications.

ASSESSMENT OF NEUROLOGIC STATUS (DISABILITY)

A rapid neurologic assessment is performed as a part of the primary trauma survey. Level of consciousness, pupillary size and reactivity, and motor response are evaluated. Alcohol and other drugs may impact on the sensorium. Injury to the CNS must be excluded as a primary reason for neurologic changes concurrent with the restoration of oxygenation and circulation. Hypoxemia and hypovolemia (secondary insults) worsen the morbidity and mortality associated with brain injury. Patients with severe head injury (GCS < 9) should undergo immediate intubation with mechanical ventilation irrespective of respiratory status at that time. Because clinical examination of the abdomen in patients with severe brain injury is not possible, abdominal ultrasound or diagnostic peritoneal lavage should be performed in the early stages of management of the hypotensive patient with apparent brain injury.

Completion of the neurologic examination is performed during the secondary survey and serial evaluations of level of consciousness are mandatory. We perform a brain CT scan in every patient with known loss of consciousness, a Glasgow coma scale score of less than 15, or evidence of significant injury above the clavicles.

COMPLETION OF ASSESSMENT AND MANAGEMENT OF TRAUMA PATIENT

Reassessment of vital signs, complete history of the mechanism of injury, past medical history, and a meticulous head-to-toe examination must be obtained in every trauma victim following an appropriate response to the initial resuscitation. Every trauma patient should be treated as if they have a "full stomach." Nasogastric or orogastric tubes should be used for stomach decompression in all patients with an altered level of consciousness, who require intubation, or have associated abdominal injuries. A urinary bladder catheter should be inserted in every patient with significant injury as part of the hemodynamic assessment, or to facilitate further diagnostic studies such as diagnostic peritoncal lavage, abdominal ultrasound, or CT scan.

Baseline laboratory tests should include only an ABG with hematocrit, and a type and cross-matching. Other laboratory tests are not useful in the typical trauma victim. Base deficit obtained as a part of blood gas analysis has considerable clinical significance. The magnitude of a metabolic acidosis has prognostic value (25). In patients with a normal GCS, mortality exceeds 50% if base deficit is more than 20 (26–28). A persistent metabolic acidosis reflects a state of ongoing hypoperfusion.

RADIOLOGIC EVALUATION

The two diagnostic radiologic studies that must be performed early in the care of the trauma patient with significant blunt trauma are the anteroposterior view of the chest and pelvis. Abdominal ultrasound has proved to be very sensitive in determining intraperitoneal as well as intrapericardiac fluid and has almost replaced the diagnostic peritoneal lavage (29,30) (picture). The limitations of ultrasound include its low sensitivity in detecting retroperitoneal injuries or hollow viscus injuries in the early stages of trauma when no intraperitoneal fluid exists. Lavage is more sensitive in detecting hollow viscus injury and diaphragmatic injuries than ultrasound, but it is more time consuming, requires special equipment and surgical skill, and has approximately a 1% major complication rate.

CT scanning is an extremely helpful diagnostic method, particularly for assessing solid organ injury and retroperitoneal injury. Organ injury scales based on CT findings combined with the patient's clinical condition permit safe, nonoperative management of some injuries. The presence of vascular "blush" (area of increased enhancement) in solid organs (picture) or pelvic vessels diagnosed by CT may be controlled by angiographic embolization (picture). CT provides sufficient information about injuries to retroperitoneal organs (pancreas, adrenals, kidneys, and retroperitoneal parts of the colon and duodenum). It is also very sensitive for the diagnosing of spine and pelvic fractures. There are two major limitations of CT scanning in trauma patients. First, unstable patients cannot be transferred to the CT room; and second, the lack of reliability in the diagnosis of hollow viscus injury.

The role of interventional radiology in the management of trauma patients is currently evolving. Spiral CT angiography has largely replaced conventional angiography in many trauma centers; however, diagnostic angiography is still the procedure of choice in many hospitals around the world. The angiographic signs of hemorrhage or vascular injury include: (i) extravasation of contrast, (ii) outpouching of the arterial wall that contains contrast, which represents the rupture of the intima and media but not adventitia of the vascular wall (pseudoaneurysm), (iii) abrupt cutoff of a vessel, and (iv) arteriovenous fistula, seen as an early filling of the venous system from an injured arterial wall. Angiography is not only an extremely sensitive diagnostic test, but can also be an excellent treatment modality. Different embolic materials are used for bleeding control in trauma patients with a high success rate. Angioplasty and stent placement can also be appropriate in the trauma patient. Partial occlusion or flow limiting dissection in situations where surgical repair is not feasible may be managed by placement of an intravascular stent with improvement of blood flow. Other imaging modalities such as MRI are still under investigation and are not routinely used in acute trauma settings.

THE MULTIPLE TRAUMA PATIENT WITH LOWER EXTREMITY INJURY: THE TRAUMA SURGEON PERSPECTIVE

The trauma surgeon must consider a few distinctive features of lower extremity trauma while taking care of multiply injured patients. These considerations include associated injuries, systemic effects of lower extremity trauma, and the place of limb injury treatment in the management algorithm of multiple trauma.

Associated Injuries

Severe lower extremity injuries suggest a high-energy mechanism of injury with frequent associated injuries (31). Concomitant vascular injuries should be suspected in specific lower extremity injuries, such as posterior knee dislocation (32). However, significant vascular injuries may also complicate blunt femur (33) and tibial fractures (34).

Hemodynamic Consequences of Lower Extremity Injuries

Open lower extremity fractures with a vessel laceration may cause significant external bleeding, usually amenable to control by direct or proximal pressure. Up to 20 mL/kg of blood can accumulate in the thigh in cases of closed femur fractures (35). Prompt immobilization and traction decreases the amount of bleeding into the soft tissues of the thigh. Isolated closed femur fractures rarely cause high-grade shock (36); however, lower extremity injuries may contribute to hemodynamic instability in multiply injured patients. Urgent surgical procedures for lower extremity injuries may be indicated after excluding injuries with a higher priority for treatment. It is essential to closely monitor these patients in the operating room by both the anesthesia team and the trauma team for the development of hypoperfusion, hypothermia, acidosis, or coagulopathy (37). When these physiological derangements occur, the operation must be rapidly terminated and the patient moved to the intensive care unit.

Systemic Complications

The large amount of soft tissue in the lower extremity may lead to a massive release of inflammatory mediators after significant limb injury. This may be associated with a higher risk for late complications, such as acute respiratory distress syndrome or multiple organ dysfunction (38).

"Compartment syndrome" is another potential systemic effect of trauma to the extremities, leading to rhabdomyolysis followed by renal dysfunction. The most common injury associated with compartment syndrome is tibial fracture. Early recognition and prompt fasciotomy are the keys to the prevention of significant morbidity and mortality (39).

"Fat emboli syndrome" classically complicates the postinjury course on the third or fourth day. Although fat embolism may occur in up to 90% of patients with long bone fractures, it causes a significant clinical syndrome in less than 5% of these patients (40,41). The CNS, lungs, and kidneys are the most commonly affected organs. The diagnosis is based on a combination of clinical evidence of organ dysfunction, presence of typical petechia, and complementary laboratory studies. Only supportive treatment is indicated. Although early long bone fixation has been thought to reduce the occurrence of fat emboli syndrome, the relationship between operative fracture fixation and the development of this syndrome remains uncertain.

Vascular damage and stasis due to immobilization predispose the trauma patient to thromboembolism, which is common after major lower extremity injuries. Indeed, long bone fracture is one of the most common injuries complicated by deep vein thrombosis (DVT) and pulmonary embolism. Sequential compression devices (SCD) are the method of choice for DVT prophylaxis in trauma patients, but anticoagulation is preferred in patients with major lower extremity injuries because SCD are ineffective when used in only a single lower extremity (unpublished data). In circumstances where both compression sleeves and anticoagulation are contraindicated, a prophylactic inferior vena cava filter should be considered.

Treatment Considerations in Multiple Trauma Patients

There are several situations in which the trauma surgeon perspective should influence the decision to operate on patients with lower extremity injuries. Early fixation of fractures is preferred today due to numerous potential benefits, such as enabling early mobilization, better pain control, and improved pulmonary toileting. However, there is little evidence that early fixation improves the outcome of trauma patients with multiple severe injuries (42). On the other hand, there is no objective data to support the theory that early fixation has deleterious effects on patients with lung injury or intracranial hypertension from head trauma (43). The timing of orthopedic surgical intervention should be individualized for each patient based on physiological status. There are cases, such as high-grade open fractures, where urgent orthopedic intervention is indicated. The hemodynamic, respiratory, and neurological status of the patient may at times dictate the length of the orthopedic procedure. Patients that develop acidosis, hypothermia, and coagulopathy, or severe respiratory insufficiency may require abbreviated operations. Application of temporary external fixation may be required until definitive internal fixation can be performed safely (44). Finally, there are rare cases in which associated injuries or physiological conditions may force the surgeon to emergently amputate a mangled limb that might have been otherwise salvaged if the patient was stable.

CONCLUSION

Devastating limb injuries may distract the treating team from more life-threatening lesions. In this chapter, we have emphasized the critical importance of adhering to the general algorithm of establishing a definitive airway and maintaining adequate respiratory function and circulation. The recognition that traumatic brain injury accounts for 50% of trauma-related deaths is essential. Secondary hypoxia and, more importantly, hypotensive insults must be avoided. The various diagnostic modalities that help in identifying injuries to the head, chest, abdomen, and pelvis must be utilized in a rapid and efficient manner while observing the patient's response to resuscitation. Finally, those patients that become hemodynamically unstable or fail to respond to resuscitation belong either in the operating room (intracavitary bleeding) or in the angiography suite (bleeding from a pelvic fracture). In cases of polytrauma with severe lower extremity injuries, the proper treatment strategy must be based upon continuous discussion between the trauma and orthopedic surgeon. This team approach will provide the multiple trauma patient with the best chance for survival.

REFERENCES

1. Fingerhut LA, Warner M. Injury Chartbook: Health, United States, 1996–1997. Hyattsville, MD: National Center for Health Statistics, 1997.
2. MacKenzie EJ, Fowler CJ. In: Mattox KL, Feliciano DV, Moore EE, eds. Epidemiology. Trauma 2000; 2:22.
3. Sauaia A, Moore FA, Moore EE, et al. Epidemiology of trauma deaths: a reassessment. J Trauma 1995; 38(2):185–193.
4. Trunkey DD. Trauma. Sci Am 1983; 249:28.
5. Cales RH, Trunkey DD. Preventable trauma deaths: a review of trauma system development. J Am Med Assoc 1985; 254(8):1059–1063.
6. American College of Surgeons Committee on Trauma: Resources for the Optimal Care of the Injured Patient. Chicago: American College of Surgeons, 1993.
7. O'Malley KF, Ross SE. The incidence of injury to the cervical spine in patients with craniocerebral injury. J Trauma 1988; 28(10):1476–1478.
8. Ross SE, Schwab CW, David ET, Delong WG, Born CT. Clearing the cervical spine: Initial radiologic evaluation. J Trauma 1987; 27(9):1055–1060.
9. Bayless P, Ray VG. Incidence of cervical spine injuries in association with blunt head trauma. Am J Emerg Med 1989; 7(2):139–142.
10. Hills MW, Deane SA. Head injury and facial injury: is there an increased risk of cervical spine injury? J Trauma 1993; 34(4):549–553; discussion 553–554.
11. Majernick TG, Bieniek R, Houston JB, Hughes HG. Cervical spine movement during orotracheal intubation. Ann Emerg Med 1986; 15(4):417–420.
12. Vukmir RB, Rinnert KJ, Krugh JW. Trauma airway management. In: Peitzman AB, Schwab CW, Yealy DM, eds. The Trauma Manual. Lippincot-Raven, 1998:91.
13. Airway and ventilatory management. In: The American college of surgeons, eds. Advanced Trauma Life Support. 6th ed. Chicago, IL: The American College of Surgeons, 1997:59–86.
14. Shearer VE, Giesecke AH. Airway management for patients with penetrating neck trauma: a retrospective study. Anesth Analg 1993; 77(6):1135–1138.
15. Standards and Guidelines for cardiopulmonary resuscitation (CPR) and emergency cardiac care (ECC). J Am Med Assoc 1980; 244:453.
16. Logan A. Use of laryngeal mask in a patient with unstable fracture of cervical spine. Anaesthesiology 1991; 46:987.
17. Pennant JH, Pace NA, Gajraj NM. Role of laryngeal mask airway in the immobile cervical spine. J Clin Anesth 1993; 5(3):226–230.
18. Berry A, Brimacombe J. Risk of aspiration with the laryngeal mask. Br J Anaesth 1994; 73(4):565–566.
19. Brantigan CO, Grow JB, Sr. Subglottic stenosis after cricothyroidotomy. Surgery 1982; 91(2):217–221.

20. Nakayama DK, Ramenofsky ML, Rowe MI. Chest injuries in childhood. Ann Surg 1989; 210(6):770–775.
21. LoCicero J, Mattox KL. Epidemiology of chest trauma. Surg Clin North Am 1989; 69:15.
22. Ciraulo DL, Elliott D, Mitchell KA, Rodriguez A. Flail chest as a marker for significant injuries. J Am Coll Surg 1994; 178(5):466–470.
23. Freedland M, Wilson RF, Bender JS, Levison MA. The management of flail chest injury: factors affecting outcome. J Trauma Inj Inf Crit Care 1990; 30(12):1460–1468.
24. Wolinsky PR. Assessment and management of pelvic fracture in the hemodynamically unstable patient. Orthop Clin North Am 1997; 28(3):321–329.
25. Siegel JH, Rivkind AI, Dalal S, Goodarzi S. Early physiologic predictors of injury severity and death in blunt multiple trauma. Arch Surg 1990; 125(4):498–508.
26. Rutherford EJ, Morris JA Jr, Reed GW, Hall KS. Base deficit stratifies mortality and determines therapy. J Trauma Inj Inf Crit Care 1992; 33(3):417–423.
27. Davis JW, Parks SN, Kaups KL, Gladen HE, O'Donnell-Nicol S. Admission base deficit predicts transfusion requirements and risk of complications. J Trauma 1996; 41(5):769–774.
28. Mizock BA, Falk JL. Lactic acidosis in critical illness. Crit Care Med 1992; 20(1):80–93.
29. Rozycki GS, Ochsner MG, Schmidt JA, et al. A prospective study of surgeon-performed ultrasound as the primary adjuvant modality for injured patient assessment. J Trauma 1995; 39(3):492–498.
30. McKenney KL, McKenney MG, Cohn SM, et al. Hemoperitoneum score helps determine need for therapeutic laparotomy. J Trauma 2001; 50(4):650–654.
31. Adili A, Bhandari M, Lachowski RJ, Kwok DC, Dunlop RB. Organ injuries associated with femoral fractures: Implications for severity of injury in motor vehicle collisions. J Trauma 1999; 46(3):386–391.
32. Gable DR, Allen JW, Richardson JD. Blunt popliteal artery injury: is physical examination alone enough for evaluation? J Trauma 1997; 43(3):541.
33. Kluger Y, Gonze MD, Paul DB, et al. Blunt vascular injury associated with closed mid-shaft femur fracture: a plea for concern. J Trauma 1994; 36(2):222–225.
34. Brinker MR, Bailey DE, Jr. Fracture healing in tibia fractures with an associated vascular injury. J Trauma 1997; 42(1):11–19.
35. Lieurance R, Benjamin JB, Rappaport WD. Blood loss and transfusion in patients with isolated femur fractures. J Orthop Trauma 1992; 6(2):175–179.
36. Ostrum RF, Verghese GB, Santner TJ. The lack of association between femoral shaft fractures and hypotensive shock. J Orthop Trauma 1993; 7(4):338–342.
37. Crowl AC, Young JS, Kahler DM, Claridge JA, Chrzanowski DS, Pomphrey M. Occult hypoperfusion is associated with increased morbidity in patients undergoing early femur fracture fixation. J Trauma 2000; 48(2):260–267.
38. Trafton PG. In: Mattox KL, Feliciano DV, Moore EE, eds. Trauma. New York, NY: McGraw-Hill, 2000:981–1009.
39. Tiwari A, Haq AI, Myint F, Hamilton G. Acute compartment syndromes. Br J Surg 2002; 89(4):397.
40. Levy D. The fat embolism syndrome: a review. Clin Orthop Res 1990; 261:281.
41. Ganong RB. Fat emboli syndrome in isolated fractures of the tibia and femur. Clin Orthop 1993; (291):208–214.

42. Jaicks RR, Cohn SM, Moller BA. Early fracture fixation may be deleterious after head injury. J Trauma 1997; 42(1):1–5.
43. Dunham MC, Bosse MJ, Clancy TV, et al. Practice management guidelines for the optimal timing of long-bone fracture stabilization in polytrauma patients: the EAST Practice Management Guidelines Work Group. J Trauma 2001; 50(5):957.
44. Nowotarski PJ, Turen CH, Brumback RJ, Scarboro JM. Conversion of external fixation to intramedullary nailing for fractures of the shaft of the femur in multiply injured patients. J Bone Joint Surg Am 2000; 82(6):781–788.

2

Lower Extremity Surgical Anatomy

Kerry Latham

Division of Plastic Surgery, Miller School of Medicine, University of Miami, Miami, Florida, U.S.A.

Marcelo Lacayo Baez

Universidad Autonoma de Guadalajara, Guadalajara, Mexico

Milton B. Armstrong

Division of Plastic Surgery, Miller School of Medicine, University of Miami, Miami, Florida, U.S.A.

Efrain Arias

Florida State University College of Medicine, Tallahassee, Florida, U.S.A.

Lower extremity trauma is a commonly seen entity for the reconstructive surgeon. Plastic and reconstructive surgeons will be required to be able to identify which structures of the lower extremity are functional or are expected to be functional and those that are absent or devitalized. Based on the deficits or deficiencies, the reconstructive surgeon will be called on to assess whether a lower extremity can be salvaged or can be reconstructed. Knowledge of the lower extremity anatomy is one of the many tools the surgeon uses to determine recommendations for limb-threatening injuries.

The purpose of this chapter is to review the anatomy of the lower extremity (thigh and leg) with particular attention to clinically relevant or commonly useful key points. The lower extremity is composed of four major parts: the pelvic

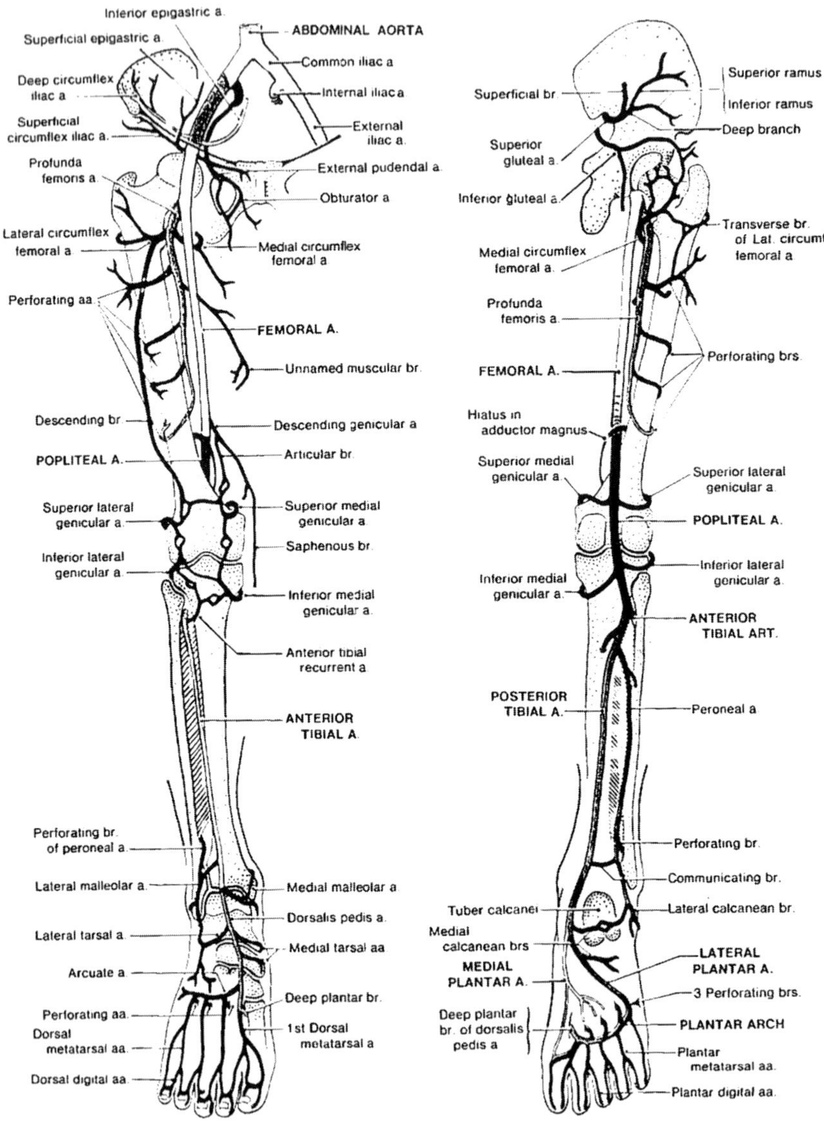

Figure 1 Vascular anatomy of the lower extremity. *Source*: From Ref. 1.

girdle, the thigh, the leg, and the foot. Only the thigh and leg will be discussed in detail in this chapter.

Embryologically the limb buds form at the fourth week of gestation on the ventrolateral aspect of the cylindrical body. By the fifth week, the limbs show regional identity, by the sixth week the hallux and rudimentary toes can be identified, and by the eighth week the toes are separated secondary to apoptosis in web spaces. By the third trimester, the limbs are well formed and nail beds are apparent.

BONY STRUCTURE

The femur carries the structural support of the lower extremity and less the tibia. The fibula is less important for weight bearing but is important for rotation (Fig. 1). The femur is the longest and strongest bone in the body. It may take up to 20 weeks to unite after fracture. The shaft is nearly cylindrical and bows forward. The distal femur flares and knuckles with two condyles articulating with the tibia. The length of the femur is associated with the length of stride and the strength is associated with the muscle mass.

The humeral head is sphenoidal with a small, rough central fovea facing anterosuperiorly to articulate with the acetabulum; the femoral neck is approximately 5 cm in length in the adult with an angle of inclination of 125° with the head. The angle of anteroversion with the shaft is 10° to 15°. The femoral head is intracapsular and alignment attaches to the fovea. The blood supply is from the medial and lateral circumflex arteries around the neck, which encircle and feed the fibrous capsule. During growth, the epiphyseal plate separates the head and neck but this fuses in maturity, and the dominant vascular supply to the head becomes the medial circumflex artery. The greater trochanter is a quadrangular projection at the junction of the neck and shaft. The proximal border is level with the center of the femoral head. The anterior surface is rough, and a flat, smooth valley divides the lateral surface. The lesser trochanter is a conical posteromedial projection at the junction of the shaft and neck. An intertrochanteric ridge descends from the superiomedial greater trochanter to the anteromedial lesser trochanter and continues distally as the spiral line. The anterior neck is intracapsular.

The posterior medial proximal shaft has a rough spiral line, and posteriolaterally has the rough gluteal tuberosity. The shaft is a cylinder of compact bone with a large medullary center. The wall is thickest in the center where the bone is the narrowest. The anterior surface is largely smooth here. The posterior surface carries the rough vertical linea aspera. The distal third of the shaft of the femur has a flat, rough posterior surface where the linea aspera widens and splays to become a rough, raised, flat projection bounded by the medial and lateral supracondylar ridges. This then becomes the triangular popliteal surface. The distal femur is widely expanded for weight bearing. The large condyles are separated by an intercondylar notch and form an articular surface with the tibia and patella, in the shape of an inverted U. The superior part of the medial condyle has a small bony prominence called the adductor tubercle. The proximal and distal femur has thinner bone and is filled with more trabecular bone with the trabeculae being disposed along the lines of stress. The femur is the first long bone to ossify after the clavicle, and it does so along five centers: shaft, head, distal, and greater and lesser trochanters. The distal femur is the only ossification center that constantly begins before birth.

The patella is the largest sesamoid bone located a little proximal to the knee joint. It has an anterior and posterior smooth surface and three borders and an apex. It is almost entirely trabecular bone covered by a thin, compact lamina. The patella ligament extends from the patella apex to the tibial tuberosity. The synovial membrane of the knee is the most complex in the entire body. There is a fibrous capsule encompassing the knee. There are four anterior, four lateral, five medial, and one posterior bursa. There are menisci, which are crescentic cartilages that probably assist in lubrication.

The proximal tibia has massive medial and lateral condyles, an intercondylar area, and a tibial tuberosity. The medial articular surface is oval and centrally concave, whereas the lateral surface is round and centrally concave. The tibial tuberosity is the apex of the anterior triangular area where the condylar surfaces merge. The anterior intercondylar area is smooth and receives the anterior cruciate ligament, whereas the posterior intercondylar area is where the posterior cruciate ligament attaches. The condyles overhang the shaft, which is triangular with medial-lateral and posterior surfaces. On the posterior surface, there is an oblique soleal line that the popliteus attaches to superiorly. Distal to the soleal line and coursing vertically is the vertical line, which separates the flexor digitorum longus (FDL) (medial) and tibialis posterior. The distal tibia expands and is laterally rotated. It has a posterior, anterior, medial, and lateral surface. The lateral surface possesses the fibular notch, which supports the interosseous membrane. The interosseous membrane has a window proximally where the anterior tibial artery (AT) penetrates anteriorly. Distally a window in the membrane exists for perforating branches of the peroneal artery. Ossification of the tibia occurs at three centers: the shaft and both epiphyses.

The fibula is a more slender long bone than the tibia and is not directly involved in weight bearing. The head is slightly expanded and connects to the tibia by a proximal synovial and distal fibrous joint. Proximally it only articulates with the tibia, but distally the fibula articulates with the tibia and the talus. Their shafts are also united by an interosseous membrane or syndesmose. The triangular area at the lateral malleolus is subcutaneous but the rest of the bone is obscured by muscles. It ossifies by three centers, two on the ends and one in the shaft. The fibula flap is a type V flap as it is supplied by nutrient endosteal and periosteal muscular and septal pedicles from the peroneal artery, which enters the fibula from posterior to the interosseous membrane 14–19 cm below the styloid process in the middle third of the fibula. The fibula flap is innervated by the superficial peroneal nerve. The fibula can be harvested with muscle or muscle and skin and from an anterior or posterior approach. When it is harvested, the peroneus muscles must be taken down. The common and superficial nerves run in close proximity to the fibula and should be avoided. Any osteotomies should be made well away from the nutrient vessel. The leg compartments are opened to release the muscular attachments to the fibula.

VASCULAR ANATOMY

Arteries of the Lower Extremity

Common Femoral Artery

The external iliac artery enters the thigh posterior to the inguinal ligament becoming the femoral artery.

The common femoral artery (CFA) is the main lower limb artery and lies posterior to the deep fascia. It corresponds to the proximal third of a line from the middle point between the anterior superior iliac spine and the pubic symphysis all the way to the adductor tubercle.

The CFA goes from the inguinal ligament to the distal border of the popliteus and then divides itself into anterior and posterior tibial arteries. The proximal part of the CFA lies among the knee extensor muscles, whereas when it reaches the popliteal area (becoming the popliteal artery) it irrigates flexor muscles.

Within the femoral triangle, the CFA is surrounded by different structures mentioned elsewhere. At the inferior end of the femoral triangle, the CFA crosses with the femoral vein becoming anterior to it. The adductor canal is another space with important surrounding structures that is mentioned elsewhere in the text.

The branches of the CFA are the following.

1. Superficial inferior epigastric artery begins anterior from the CFA and 1 cm from the inguinal ligament, and ascends with it anteriorly. It supplies the superficial inguinal lymph nodes and the superficial fascia and skin. It anastomoses with branches from the inferior epigastric artery.

2. Superficial circumflex iliac artery begins near the superficial epigastric artery through the fascia lata, and lateral to the opening of the saphenous vein turns laterally from the inguinal ligament moving toward the anterior superior iliac spine. It supplies skin, superficial fascia, and superficial inguinal lymph nodes. It anastomoses with the deep circumflex iliac and lateral circumflex iliac artery.

3. Superficial external pudendal artery arises medial to the CFA from the cribiform fascia. It passes deep to the saphenous vein and across the spermatic cord to supply lower abdominal, penile, scrotal, or labial skin.

4. Deep external pudendal artery trajectory is medial crossing the pectineus and anterior or posterior to the adductor longus. It is covered by the fascia lata, and it pierces it to irrigate the skin of the perineum, scrotum, or labium majus.

5. Muscular branches supply sartorius, vastus medialis, and adductor muscles.

Arteria Profunda Femoris

This is the main thigh artery and the largest branch of the CFA, and then it spirals posterior to it and to the femoral vein locating itself on the femoral medial side. As it leaves the femoral triangle, it travels between the pectineus and the adductor longus and between the adductor longus and the adductor brevis continuing between the adductor longus and the adductor magnus. The profunda pierces through the adductor magnus and anastomoses with the upper muscular branches of the popliteal artery.

This final part is called the fourth perforating artery, and it is simply the terminal end of the profunda. The profunda is the main blood supply to the extensor muscles, adductor muscles, and flexor muscles.

The branches of the profunda are as follow.

The lateral and medial circumflex femoral arteries supply the lateral thigh muscles and the proximal end of the femur.

1. Lateral circumflex femoral artery (LCFA) divides itself into ascending, descending, and transverse branches. The ascending branch is lateral to the hip joint and along the intertrochanteric line. It anastomoses with the superior gluteal and deep circumflex iliac arteries, and supplies the greater trochanter. It forms an anastomotic ring around the femoral neck with the medial circumflex femoral artery (MCFA) supplying the femoral neck and head. The descending branch descends posterior to the rectus femoris passing along the anterior border of the vastus lateralis supplying it. Within vastus lateralis, a long branch descends toward the knee, and this branch anastomoses with the lateral superior genicular branch of the popliteal. The transverse branch is the smaller one and it passes lateral and anterior to the vastus intermedius. It pierces vastus lateralis and circles around the femur distal to the greater trochanter. It anastomoses with the medial circumflex, inferior gluteal, and first perforating arteries, called cruciate anastomosis.

2. MCFA supplies the adductor muscles and curves between pectineus and psoas major around the femur. It appears between the quadratus femoris and upper border of the adductor magnus. Here it divides into transverse and ascending branches. The transverse branch forms part of the cruciate anastomosis. The ascending branch goes to the tendon of the obturator externus, anterior to the quadratus femoris. It anastomoses with branches of the gluteal and the LCFA. There is also an acetabular branch that enters the hip joint under the transverse acetabular ligament along with a branch from the obturator artery. It supplies the fossa fat and the femoral head.

3. The perforating arteries — perforators are usually three and pass deep within the iliopsoas and pectineus to the posterior of the thigh being the major suppliers of blood to the head and neck of the femur. The first perforator travels between the pectineus and the adductor brevis, pierces the adductor magnus to supply adductor brevis, adductor magnus, biceps femoris, and gluteus maximus. It anastomoses with the inferior gluteal, MCFA, LCFA, and second perforator. The second perforator arises with the first perforator and divides into ascending and descending branches to supply the posterior femoral muscles and anastomoses with the first and third perforators. The femoral nutrient artery arises from the second perforator, but when two of these exist they usually arise from the first and third perforators. The third perforator begins distally to the adductor brevis and pierces through the attachment of adductor magnus going to the posterior femoral muscles. Its proximal anastomosis is with the perforators, its distal anastomosis is the terminal branch of the profunda (fourth perforator) and the muscular branches of the popliteal.

4. Muscular branches arise from the profunda and end in the adductor muscles; some pierce into the adductor magnus, and still others supply the flexor muscles. They anastomose with the MCFA and superior muscular popliteal branches.

There is an anastomotic formation in the back of the thigh that supplies from the gluteal region to the popliteal fossa formed proximodistally by:

- Gluteal arteries and terminals of the MCFA,
- LCFA, MCFA, and the first perforator,
- Perforators and each other,

- Fourth perforator (terminal end of the profunda) and superior muscular branches of the popliteal.

Descending Genicular Artery

The descending genicular artery arises from the CFA proximal to the adductor magnus's hiatus. It has three branches: saphenous, articular, and muscular.

1. The saphenous branch of the descending genicular artery emerges distally to the adductor magnus's hiatus, accompanies the saphenous nerve to the medial side of the knee, and passes between the sartorius and gracilis. It supplies the skin of the proximomedial area of the leg. The branch anastomoses with the medial inferior genicular artery.

2. The muscular branches arise proximal to the adductor magnus's hiatus and descend in the vastus medialis anterior to the adductor magnus's tendon. Then they move to the side of the knee and anastomose with the medial superior genicular artery. Both the vastus medialis and the adductor magnus are supplied by the muscular branches, which give off the articular branches.

3. These articular branches anastomose on the knee joint. One articular branch crosses above the femoral patellar surface and forms an arch with the lateral superior genicular artery, supplying the knee joint.

Popliteal Artery

The popliteal begins distal to the hiatus of the adductor magnus and it descends to the intercondylar fossa, finally inclines laterally and divides into AT and posterior tibial artery (PT) at the inferior border of the popliteus muscle at the crural interosseous space. Anterior to the popliteal is the fat on the posterior part of the femur, the fibrous capsule of the knee joint, and the popliteus fascia. On the posterior side of the popliteal are the semimembranosus muscle, popliteal vein, tibial nerve, and gastrocnemius muscle. The lateral side of the popliteal contains the biceps femoris, tibial nerve, popliteal vein, lateral femoral condyle, the plantaris, and lateral heads of the gastrocnemius. Finally, the medial side of the popliteal contains the semimembranosus muscle, medial femoral condyle, tibial nerve, popliteal vein, and the medial head of the gastrocnemius.

The branches of the popliteal are as follow.

1. The cutaneous branches, which descend between the head of the gastrocnemius, and perforate the deep fascia to supply the skin on the back of the leg.

2. The superior muscular branches, which are two or three, and pass to adductor magnus and femoral flexors and finally anastomose with the fourth popliteal or the terminal end of the Profunda.

3. The sural arteries, which are two, and are behind the knee joint supplying the gastrocnemius, soleus, and plantaris muscles; the superior genicular arteries, which arise from the popliteal and curve around, proximal to both femoral condyles to the anterior area of the knee. Smaller branches of the superior genicular arteries are also relevant.

The medial superior genicular artery travels under the semimembranosus and semitendinosus, proximal to the medial head of the gastrocnemius, and deeply to the adductor magnus's tendon. It gives branches to the vastus medialis and anastomoses superiorly with the deep genicular artery, inferiorly with the medial inferior genicular artery and finally ramifies on the femur and unites with the lateral superior genicular artery.

The lateral superior genicular artery passes under the tendon of the biceps femoris and then divides into superior and deep branches. The superior branch supplies the vastus lateralis and anastomoses superiorly with the LCFA, inferiorly with the lateral inferior genicular artery, and deeply with the medial superior genicular artery forming an arch across the femur that unites with the descending genicular artery.

4. The middle genicular artery is another branch of the popliteal that arises from the posterior center of the knee joint, pierces the oblique popliteal ligament, and supplies the cruciate ligaments and synovial membrane of the knee.

5. The inferior genicular artery goes deep to the gastrocnemius from the popliteal and has medial and lateral branches. The medial inferior genicular artery travels deep to the medial head of the gastrocnemius and descends along the proximal margin of the popliteal fossa supplying it. It passes inferior to the medial tibial condyle and under the tibial collateral ligament and finally ascends to the knee joint and supplies it. It anastomoses with the lateral inferior genicular artery, the medial superior genicular artery, and the anterior tibial recurrent artery. The lateral inferior genicular artery crosses laterally along the popliteal fossa and anastomoses with the medial inferior genicular artery and lateral superior genicular artery, the anterior tibial recurrent and posterior tibial recurrent arteries, and finally the circumflex fibular arteries.

In this area of the knee, there exists an important genicular anastomosis made up of the following arteries: medial genicular arteries, lateral genicular arteries, descending genicular artery, descending branch of the LCFA, circumflex fibular artery, and finally anterior tibial recurrent artery and posterior tibial recurrent artery.

Anterior Tibial Artery

The AT arises at the distal end of the popliteal fossa as the terminal branch of the popliteal. It is initially located in the flexor compartment and then goes posteriorly through the oval aperture in the proximal part of the interosseous membrane to the extensor region, medial to the fibular neck. At the ankle it is midway between the malleoli, continuing on the dorsal part of the foot as the arteria dorsalis pedis.

In the proximal two-thirds of its trajectory, it is on the interosseous membrane, and in the distal one-third it is anterior to the tibia all the way to the ankle joint. At this point, it is crossed by the tendon of the extensor hallucis longus (EHL). The deep peroneal nerve reaches the lateral side of the AT as it enters the extensor compartment, becomes anterior to it in the middle third of the leg, and once again lateral in the last third of the leg.

The AT is found approximately 2.5 cm distal to the medial side of the fibular head. It ends midway between the malleoli.

The branches of the AT are as follow.

1. The posterior tibial recurrent artery arises before the AT reaches the extensor compartment. It supplies the superior tibiofibular joint.

2. The anterior tibial recurrent artery, which is born close to the posterior tibial recurrent artery, then ascends in tibialis anterior ramifying on the front and side of the knee joint.

3. The muscular branches, which supply the adjacent muscles, some also the skin, and some anastomosing with the posterior tibial and peroneal arteries.

4. The anterior medial malleolar artery, which is born 5 cm proximal to the ankle, posterior to the EHL's tendons.

5. The anterior lateral malleolar artery, which travels posterior to the tendons of the extensor digitorum longus (EDL) to the lateral side of the ankle.

The ankle joint anastomoses consist of a vascular network around the malleoli. The medial malleolar network is made up of: (1) the anterior medial malleolar branch of the AT; (2) medial tarsal branches of the arteria dorsalis pedis; (3) the malleolar and calcaneal branches of the PT; and (4) branches of the medial plantar artery. The lateral malleolar network is made up of: (1) the anterior lateral malleolar branch of the AT; (2) the lateral tarsal branch of arteria dorsalis pedis; (3) the perforating calcaneal branches of the peroneal; and (4) side branches of the lateral plantar artery. The AT becomes the arteria dorsalis pedis at the ankle joint level.

The tibial peroneal trunk is the arterial section between the AT and the PT distal to the popliteal and proximal to the PT.

Posterior Tibial Artery

The PT arises from the distal border of the popliteal fossa between the tibia and the fibula. As it descends down the leg, it is located in the flexor muscles' compartment. It divides between the medial malleolus and the medial tubercle of calcaneus into medial and lateral plantar arteries.

The PT has the following branches.

1. The circumflex fibular artery passes on a lateral path around the fibula's neck going through the soleus muscle anastomosing then with the lateral inferior genicular artery, medial genicular arteries, and anterior tibial recurrent artery. It supplies both bone and articulation.

2. The peroneal artery arises distal to the popliteal fossa passing in an oblique direction to the fibula, and descending then by its medial crest between tibialis posterior and flexor hallucis longus (FHL). Once it reaches the inferior tibiofibular syndesmosis, it divides into calcaneal branches. Proximally covered by soleus and deep transverse fascia, and distally overlapped by FHL, it also gives off some muscular branches that supply the soleus, tibialis posterior, FHL, and peronei.

3. The nutrient artery of the tibia, which is born from the PT at its origin, descending into the bone immediately after the soleal line. Its muscular branches supply the soleus and the deep leg flexors. The communicating branch of the posterior tibia runs posterior to the tibia and across it, approximately 5 cm superior to its distal end. It lies deep to the FHL. It joins a communicating peroneal

artery branch. The medial malleolar branches pass around the tibial malleolus and go to the medial malleolar network.

Veins of the Lower Extremities

Superficial Veins of the Lower Extremities

The great saphenous vein is the body's longest vein coming off of the medial marginal vein and heading upward toward the femoral vein where it ends a short distance away from the inguinal ligament. It ascends about 3 cm anterior to the medial malleolus, then crosses medially the distal end of the tibia obliquely to the medial border, then ascends again to the knee. Around the knee it is located posteromedial to the femoral and medial tibial condyles, at which point it ascends the medial thigh. It finally joins to the femoral vein after crossing the saphenous opening. Branches of the medial femoral cutaneous nerve travel with the great saphenous vein throughout its course in the thigh. The saphenous branch of the descending genicular artery (at the knee) and the saphenous nerve (in foot and leg) are both anterior to the vein. It contains about 10 to 20 valves, one located just before it pierces the cribiform fascia and another at its union with the femoral vein. The valves are more frequent in the leg than in the thigh. The vein contains connections with the deep veins (mostly in the leg region) and lies in the superficial fascia throughout most of its length.

Tributaries

Medial marginal veins that lead into the great saphenous vein at the ankle drain the sole of the foot. In the leg, perforating veins connect it with deep veins and with small saphenous veins. Distal to the knee there are normally three tributaries: one from the calf, another from the front of the leg, and third from the tibial malleolar region, which forms below in a fine network of veins over the medial malleolus and then ascends over the medial region of the calf as the posterior crural arch vein. Perforating vcins join the great saphenous vein at two main sites. One is at the area of the upper calf by the tibial tubercle perforator, and the other is the Hunterian perforator in the lower third of the thigh.

Many tributaries are received by the great saphenous vein in the thigh. Some form large named channels that often pass the base of the femoral triangle before connecting with the great saphenous near its union with the femoral vein while others open independently. These can be grouped as anterolateral tributaries (one or more), posteromedial tributaries (one or more), and peri-inguinal veins (four or more). The anterior femoral cutaneous vein (anterolateral vein of the thigh) usually starts from an anterior network of veins in the distal thigh and crosses the distal half and apex of the femoral triangle to meet with the great saphenous vein. As the anterior femoral cutaneous vein crosses the saphenous opening, it is joined by superficial circumflex iliac (drain anterior abdominal wall) and superficial external pudendal veins (drain the scrotum) along with the superficial epigastric vein (drain anterior abdominal wall). The posteriomedial vein of the thigh drains a large superficial region of the same name. Sometimes it is called the accessory saphenous vein when there are more than one posteromedial branch present, referring to the lowest vein.

The lesser saphenous vein begins as a continuation of the lateral marginal veins posterior to the lateral malleolus. It ascends lateral to the tendo calcaneus in the lower third of the calf. By the midline of the calf medially it penetrates into the deep fascia where it ascends on the gastrocnemius. It passes between the heads of the gastrocnemius as it continues to ascend until it reaches its destination at the popliteal vein in the popliteal fossa, 3–7.5 cm above the knee joint. The lesser saphenous vein sends a few rami medially and proximally to join the great saphenous vein while receiving many cutaneous tributaries in the leg. It also unites with deep veins on the dorsum of the foot. It contains about 7 to 13 valves. Its termination is variable; it can bifurcate, one branch joining the popliteal or deep posterior femoral vein, and the other joining the great saphenous vein; it can just unite in the thigh with the great saphenous; it can also terminate in the deep sural muscular or great saphenous vein distal to the knee.

Clinical note: Venous return from the lower limb is largely dependent on contraction of the calf muscles, also known as the "calf pump," which is aided by the tight sleeve of deep fascia. The great saphenous and the deep veins are connected by perforating veins, especially near the ankle, knee, and distal calf region. Valves in these channels prevent flow of blood from deep to superficial veins. Upon contraction of the calf muscles, blood is pumped proximally in the deep veins and at the same time the valves in the perforating veins prevent it from entering the superficial veins. If the valves become incompetent in the perforating veins, it can lead to high-pressure leaks during contractions of the muscle. The dilation of superficial veins can result in varicosities, anoxia, and eventually varicose ulcerations.

Deep Veins of the Lower Extremities

Posterior tibial veins travel along with the PT and receive veins from the venous plexus in soleus, peroneal veins, and connections from superficial veins, which are all located in the sural muscles.

Anterior tibial veins exit the extensor region between the fibula and the tibia, pass through the proximal part of the interosseous membrane, and eventually come together with the posterior tibial veins at the distal region of the popliteus to form the popliteal vein. They are the venous continuation of the vessel that accompanies the dorsal pedal artery.

The popliteal vein eventually becomes the femoral vein after passing through the adductor hiatus and ascending into the popliteal fossa. It is located medial to the artery distally; it is superficial to the artery between the heads of the gastrocnemius muscle; and it is posterolateral to the artery proximally to the knee joint. It contains four valves and its tributaries are the venous branches of the partners to the popliteal artery, muscular veins, and the small saphenous vein.

The femoral vein begins at the adductor hiatus as the continuation of the popliteal, and ends as the external iliac posterior to the inguinal ligament. It is posterolateral to the femoral artery, which it accompanies in the adductor canal distally; proximally in the canal and also in the femoral triangle distally (apex) it is located posterior to the artery; at the base of the triangle it is located medial to the artery. Between the femoral artery and the canal, the vein is located in the femoral sheath in the middle compartment. The venus profunda femoris unites with it posteriorly about 4–12 cm distal to the inguinal ligament and then anteriorly the greater saphenous vein joins it. Medial and lateral circumflex femoral veins also contribute to it. Normally it contains four to five valves, with one near the inguinal ligament and another being distal to the joining of the profunda femoris.

The profunda femoral vein has a few tributaries through which it unites proximally with the inferior gluteal veins and distally with the popliteal veins. It is located anterior to its artery. It has a valve just before it terminates and drains lateral and medial circumflex femoral veins.

LYMPHATIC DRAINAGE

Lymphatic Drainage of the Lower Extremities

Superficial inguinal nodes form distal and proximal groups. About four to five nodes from the distal group are usually found along the termination of the great saphenous vein. These nodes receive mostly all superficial vessels of the lower extremities except those coming from the calf's region posterolaterally. Through the femoral canal and also anteriorly or laterally to the femoral vessels, all superficial inguinal lymph nodes drain to the external iliac nodes. Just distal to the inguinal ligament about five to six from the proximal group are found. Its medial members receive superficial vessels from external genitalia, perianal region, inferior anal canal, umbilicus, abdominal wall, and uterine vessels. Lateral members receive afferent vessels from anterior abdominal wall inferior to the umbilicus and the gluteal region.

Deep inguinal nodes are situated medially to the femoral vein varying from three to five. One is in the femoral canal, another is located distally to the saphenofemoral junction; the most proximal one in the femoral ring lies laterally. Cloquet's node is the most superior node located under the inguinal ligament. Normally surgeons use this node to figure out whether the cancer has metastasized further into the deep compartments. They all receive deep lymph vessels that accompany the femoral artery and vein, lymphatics from the glans of the clitoris (or penis), and some efferent vessels from the superficial inguinal lymph nodes; their own efferents reach the external iliac nodes by crossing the femoral canal.

Popliteal lymph nodes are usually six small nodes that are embedded in popliteal fat. One is between the posterior aspect of the knee joint and the popliteal artery receiving afferent vessels accompanying the genicular arteries and direct vessels from the knee joint. Another is located near the end of the small saphenous vein and drains the superficial area drained by the vein. The popliteal vessels are flanked by the nodes that are left, which receive afferent trunks traveling along with the anterior and posterior tibial vessels. Efferents of popliteal nodes ascend to reach the deep inguinal nodes by traveling close to the femoral vessels mostly, but there are also some that ascend close to the great saphenous vein and head toward the superficial inguinal nodes.

Superficial Tissue Lymph Drainage in Lower Limbs

The subcutaneous plexus is where the superficial lymph vessels are derived from. Lymph vessels leave the foot both laterally along the lesser saphenous vein and along the great saphenous medially.

Lateral vessels cross anteriorly in the leg and join the medial vessels to head toward the distal superficial inguinal lymph nodes; others head toward the popliteal nodes by traveling along the small saphenous vein. In the gluteal region, superficial lymph vessels circle anteriorly and head to the proximal superficial inguinal nodes. The medial vessels begin at the foot's dorsum on the tibial side and they are more numerous and larger. These vessels ascend both anteriorly and posteriorly to the medial malleolus; both eventually converging on the great saphenous vein and traveling with it to the distal superficial inguinal nodes.

Deep Tissue Lymph Drainage in Lower Limbs

Anterior and posterior tibial, popliteal, peroneal, and femoral vessels are all followed by deep lymph vessels. The deep lymph vessels in the leg and foot head toward the popliteal nodes and those that are located in the thigh head toward the deep inguinal nodes.

The deep lymph vessels have their correspondent blood vessels, which they follow, in the ischial and gluteal region. Lymph vessels following the inferior gluteal vessels cross one or two small nodes inferior to the piriformis and head toward the internal iliac nodes.

Clinical note: Enlargement of the superficial inguinal lymph nodes frequently occurs and is due to injury or disease in their region of drainage. Lateral lesions in the heel often lead to inflammation of the popliteal nodes.

FASCIA AND COMPARTMENTS

The leg covered in superficial fascia under the subcutaneous tissue is made of loose connective tissue and is continuous with scarpa's fascia. In certain areas, this superficial fascia splits into two layers to accommodate the passage of superficial vessels such as the lesser saphenous vein, greater saphenous vein, and superficial inguinal lymph nodes. The femoral sheath, which is an extension of deep abdominal wall fascia (transversalis and iliacus) is continuous with the cribiform fascia, which makes up the deep fascia of the thigh in the area of the saphenous opening. The greater saphenous vein perforates this in the proximal thigh to enter the femoral vein here. The deep fascia of the thigh or fascia lata is a strong, broad, thick layer that invests the thigh muscles. It encases the tensor fascia lata muscle and is thickened laterally contributing to the iliotibial tract. In the leg the deep fascia is called the crural fascia. It does not completely invest all the muscles; instead it is attached to the anterior and medial borders of the tibia and is contiguous with the periosteum. The crural fascia is thick proximally and laterally it thins distally but thickens again to form the superior and inferior retinaculum. The superior extensor retinaculum passes from the fibular to the tibia, and it binds the extensor tendons to prevent bow stringing. The Y-shaped inferior extensor retinaculum attaches laterally to the calcaneus and keeps the peroneus and EDL in position. The compartments of the leg are divided by the interosseous membrane, the crural intermuscular septum, and the tibia and fibula.

There are three compartments of the thigh: anterior, medial, and posterior. There are four compartments of the leg: anterior, lateral, superficial posterior, and deep posterior. Compartment syndrome is characterized by increased pressure within these fascial compartments generally greater than 30 mmHg or with symptoms of pain with passive motion, paresthesia or pal-or, poikilothermia, pulselessness, and paralysis in later phases. The anterior leg compartment is the most susceptible to compartment syndrome, in part due to fracture patterns, less forgiving fascial and bony constraints, and decreased collaterals from other vessels. If compartment syndrome is suspected in the leg, four-compartment fasciotomy should be performed rapidly.

The contents of each compartment are listed below:

1. Thigh
   Anterior: tensor fascia lata, sartorius, quadriceps femoris, iliacus, psoas, superficial femoral artery (SFA), and saphenous nerve.
   Medial: pectineus, gracilis, adductor magnus, adductor brevis, adductor longus, obturator, profundus femoris artery, deep saphenous vein, and obturator nerve.
   Posterior: semitendinosus, semimembranosus, biceps femoris, and sciatic nerve.
2. Leg
   Anterior: tibialis anterior, EHL, EDL, peroneus tertius muscle, anterior tibial vessels (one artery and paired veins), and deep peroneal nerve.
   Lateral: peroneus brevis (PB), peroneus longus (PL), and superficial peroneal nerve.
   Superficial deep: gastrocnemius, soleus, and plantaris.
   Deep posterior: tibialis posterior, FHL, peroneal vessels, posterior tibial vessels, tibial nerve, and FDL.

MUSCLES OF THE THIGH AND LEG

Most anatomy references group the muscles by compartment as we discuss here; however, it is also important to organize the muscle by function and circulation, which is more important for reconstruction. For example, the thigh has three compartments; however, more importantly it has three regions from which useful flaps can be harvested based on function, location, and circulation. For example, the medial groups of anatomic flaps are based largely on the superficial femoral artery, and the gracilis muscle or myocutaneous flap is the work-horse of this region. In the lateral thigh, the anteriolateral thigh flap, tensor fascia lata flap, and subtotal thigh flaps that are based on the lateral circumflex system are the work-horse flaps. Posteriorly, flaps are based on the inferior gluteal system and include the posterior thigh flap. Other muscle groups will either be too easily devascularized or loss of function is generally prohibitive. Similarly in the leg, due to the size of the muscles in the superficial deep compartment, the gastrocnemius and soleus are the work-horses of the lower leg; however, the angiosome concept becomes increasingly important in the leg and foot as, e.g., in the sural artery flap and medial and lateral plantar artery flaps.

The lower extremities consist of many intricate parts that make up its gross anatomical structure. In general, muscles, bones, arteries, veins, nerves, and the lymphatic system all play an important part. There are three bones in the leg: the femur, tibia, and fibula. The femur articulates proximally with the hip bone and distally with the tibia. The bones of the leg that join to the foot are the tibia and fibula. Connective tissue sheets divide the thigh into three compartments: anterior, medial, and posterior.

Anterior Thigh Muscles

Also known as the extensors, they cover the anterior portion of the thigh. They consist of the following muscles.

Sartorius is a muscle that is superficial, narrow, and strap-like with a slight S shape to it. It is considered to be the longest muscle in the body, which measures $5 \times 40\ cm^2$. Sometimes, it is absent. It originates at the superior iliac spine and passes across the upper and anterior part of the thigh diagonally from the lateral to the medial side of the thigh, while descending vertically to the medial side of the knee. It passes behind the medial condyle of the femur to end in a broad aponeurosis along with the gracilis and semitendinosus to form the pes anserinus and inserts on the superior part of the medial tibial condyle. It is considered to be a type IV expendable muscle that allows a person to cross the legs by flexion of the leg and lateral rotation of the thigh. The sartorius muscle is innervated by the femoral nerve and its blood supply is derived from six to seven branches off of the superficial femoral artery and vein.

The quadriceps consists of four muscles, which are the rectus femoris, vastus medialis, vastus lateralis, and vastus intermedius. These all have a common insertion on the patella, and through the patellar ligament to the tibial tuberosity of the femur.

Rectus femoris has two tendons. It originates at the anterior inferior iliac spine and superior margin of acetabulum to then insert on the patella. It is considered to be a type II and measures $20 \times 8\ cm^2$. It is a superficial muscle that is the center of the quadriceps extensor group and extends between the ilium and the patella of the knee between the vastus medialis and vastus lateralis muscles. Its actions allow for extension of the leg and some flexion of thigh. Its use as a muscle flap can result in loss of terminal leg extension, so it is not considered an expendable muscle. The superior muscle belly is innervated by the muscular branch of the femoral nerve, which supplies motor deep to the medial surface. It is also innervated by the intermediate anterior femoral cutaneous nerve (L2–3), which supplies sensory. The superior one-third of the muscle gets its major blood supply from the descending branch of the LCFA, and the superior one-fourth of the muscle gets blood supply from the ascending branch of the LCFA (both branches are off of the profunda femoral artery). The inferior one-third of the muscle gets blood from muscular branches of the superficial femoral artery.

Vastus medialis originates at the intertrochanteric line, medial lip of the linea aspera of the femur, medial proximal supracondylar line, tendons of adductor magnus, and adductor longus muscles, and medial intermuscular septum to insert on the quadriceps tendon. It is considered a type II and measures $15 \times 8\ cm^2$. This muscle is found medial to the rectus femoris and deep to the sartorius on the medial aspect of the thigh. Its action is to extend the knee, which is supported by the quadriceps group. Motor innervation is derived from the femoral nerve, whereas sensory comes from the saphenous nerve (L3–4). Its main blood supply comes from a branch of the superficial femoral artery, which enters the muscle along with the femoral nerve in the upper portion of the muscle. Some other minor branches of the superficial femoral artery run medial and deep to the muscle. Musculoarticular branches of the descending genicular artery (off of SFA) also perforate the deep to distal area of the muscle.

Vastus lateralis originates at the intertrochanteric line, greater trochanter, gluteal tuberosity, and lateral intermuscular septum to then insert on the patella. It is a type I and measures $10 \times 26\ cm^2$. This muscle is the largest in the quadriceps group extensor. It is found between the biceps femoris and the vastus intermedius muscles and beneath the tensor fascia lata, it extends from the proximal femur to the patella. Its action is to extend the leg, and because there are three other extensors in the quadriceps extensor group it is considered expendable. Motor innervation is supplied by a muscular branch of the femoral nerve, which enters at the medial border of the proximal belly adjacent and inferior to the descending branch of LCFA, while sensory is supplied by the lateral femoral cutaneous nerve (L2–3). Blood is supplied to the superior one-third of this muscle by the descending branch of LCFA (major blood supply), the superior one-fourth deep surface is penetrated by the transverse branch of the LCFA (LCFA is off of the profunda femoral artery), and the inferior one-half of the posterior muscle by posterior branches of the profunda. Also, blood is supplied to the distal muscle by a superficial branch of the lateral superior genicular artery off of the popliteal artery, which courses deep to the bicep femoris around the lateral condyle of the knee.

Vastus intermedius originates at the anterior and lateral surfaces of the upper two-thirds of the femur and from the lower part of the lateral intermuscular septum. Its fibers terminate as an aponeurosis, which forms the deep part of the quadriceps tendon and is attached to the lateral condyle of the tibia and lateral border of the patella. Its actions are involved in extension of the leg or knee. This muscle is innervated by the femoral nerve (L2–4). Blood to the vastus intermedius is supplied by the femoral artery, profunda femoral artery, and transverse and descending branches of the LCFA. Also, it gets some blood supply from the genicular branches that anastamose around the knee.

Medial Thigh Muscles

These muscles are also known as adductors of the thigh. They originate mostly from the pubis and insert on the posterior femur. They consist of the following muscles.

Pectineus originates at the pectineal line, the fascia covering the anterior surface of the muscle, and from the bone in front of it between the tubercle of the pubis and the iliopectineal eminence. The fibers pass posterolaterally to a line that goes from the lesser trochanter to the linea aspera. Its actions are adduction and flexion of the hip (thigh). Sometimes it can be attached to the hip joint. The femoral vessels and the great saphenous vein are separated from the muscle by the fascia lata, which is anterior to it. Psoas major and the medial femoral circumflex vessels lie laterally to it while the adductor longus lies medially. It is innervated by the femoral nerve (L2–3). Blood supply is derived from the obturator artery, MCFA, first perforating branch of the profunda, femoral artery, and deep external pudendal artery.

Adductor longus originates between the crest and symphysis at the pubic bone and inserts on the linea aspera. This large, fan-shaped muscle is the most superficial muscle out of the three adductors. It expands into a broad belly, which descends posterolaterally and inserts into the linea aspera of the femur between the other two adductors and vastus medialis. The spermatic cord, fascia lata, and the femoral vessels are all anterior to the muscle. Posterior to the muscle there are the other two adductor muscles, anterior branch of the obturator nerve, and the profunda femoral vessels. Gracilis is medial to the muscle while pectineus is lateral to it. Its action is adduction of the hip (thigh) and some lateral rotation. It is innervated by the anterior division of the obturator nerve. It gets its blood supply via the femoral artery, profunda femoral artery (direct and perforating branches), MCFA, and obturator artery.

Adductor brevis originates at the inferior pubic ramus and inserts on the pectineal line and linea aspera of the femur (upper posterior part of the femur). The muscle is sort of triangular in shape, and as it descends posterolaterally it expands as it heads down to the insertion site. Out of the three adductors, this is the smallest. Anteriorly there is the adductor longus, pectineus, profunda femoral artery, and anterior branch of the obturator nerve. Posteriorly is adductor magnus and posterior branch of obturator nerve. Below it there is adductor magnus and gracilis while above it there is the conjoined tendon of psoas major and iliacus, obturator externus, and MCFA. Its action is adduction of the hips (thigh) and some lateral rotation. This muscle is innervated by the obturator nerve (L2–3). It gets its blood supply via femoral artery, profunda femoral artery (first to third perforating arteries), obturator artery, and MCFA.

Adductor magnus originates at the rami of pubis and ischium, and ischial tuberosity. It then inserts on the linea aspera, medial supracondylar line (adductor part), and adductor tubercle of the femur (hamstring part). This triangular muscle is the largest of the adductor muscles and is seen from posterior view of the thigh as well. The medial part of the muscle is a thick mass that descends and ends in a round tendon in the lower third of the thigh. The long, linear attachment of the muscle has a series of openings that have tendinous arches attached to the bone. The upper four openings are small and allow perforating branches to pass through them, while the lowest one is a larger opening called the adductor hiatus formed by the tendon splitting distally allowing the femoral vessels to pass through to the popliteal fossa.

Its action is adduction of the hip (thigh) and to help control posture. It has two parts to it: the adductor part flexes the thigh, and hamstring part extends the thigh. Anterior to the muscle there is the adductor brevis and longus, pectineus, femoral, and profunda vessels. Posterior to it is the sciatic nerve, biceps femoris, semitendinosus, semimembranosus, and gluteus maximus. Medially there is the gracilis, sartorius, and fascia lata, while superiorly it is parallel with the quadratus femoris and the tranverse branch of the MCFA, which passes between the muscles. It is innervated by the obturator nerve and the tibial division of the sciatic nerve (L2–4), both nerves being from the anterior division of the lumbar plexus.

Its blood supply is derived via the femoral artery, profunda femoral artery (direct branches and all perforating arteries), obturator artery, and MCFA.

The gracilis muscle originates at the pubis symphysis and inserts at the medial tibial condyle. This thin, flat muscle that extends between the pubis and the medial knee is a type II that measures $6 \times 24\ cm^2$ and lies between the sartorius and the adductor longus muscles anteriorly and the semimembranosus posteriorly. It is considered an expendable muscle because of the presence of the adductor magnus and longus muscles. Its actions are adduction of the hip (thigh) and flexion of the leg with some medial rotation. Located between the adductor magnus and the longus muscles is the anterior branch of the obturator nerve that supplies motor and enters the deep medial surface of the gracilis muscle immediately superior to where the ascending branch of MCFA perforates it. Sensory innervation to the majority of the medial thigh is derived from the anterior femoral cutaneous nerve (L2–3). The area of skin superior to the gracilis muscle is innervated by a small cutaneous branch of the obturator nerve. The major blood supply to the superior one-third of the muscle belly is derived from the ascending branch of the MCFA off of the profunda, and the inferior one-third of the muscle gets its source from branches of the superficial femoral artery.

Posterior Thigh Muscles

This group consists only of three muscles, which are the biceps femoris, semitendinosus, and semimembranosus muscle. As a group they are referred to as the hamstring muscles. They all originate at the ischial tuberosity with the exception of the short head of the biceps femoris. The hamstrings as a group measure $15 \times 45\ cm^2$. These muscles are useful for ischial pressure sores. All the muscles of the hamstring are innervated by the same nerves. Branches of the sciatic nerve supply it with motor innervation while the postcutaneous nerve of the thigh (S1–3) supplies sensory.

Biceps femoris has two parts to it, a short and long head. This is the only muscle of the thigh that inserts laterally on the leg. The short head is mostly hidden by the long head. The two heads form a common belly and eventually have a common attachment distally. The long head originates at the ischial tuberosity and inserts on the lateral side of the head of the fibula. It is a type II muscle and measures $7 \times 10\ cm^2$. Actions of this muscle are flexion of the leg and extension of the thigh. The short head originates at the linea aspera and lateral supracondylar line of the femur and inserts at the same spot as the long head; they share the same tendon. This muscle is not expendable, because it is a strong flexor of the leg. The major artery of the long head is the first perforating branch of the profunda femoral artery, which is found at the medial aspect of the muscle. Other arteries of the muscle are the second branch of the profunda, which supplies the lower portion of the muscle medially and the inferior gluteal artery at the muscle's origin. The second or third perforating branches of the profunda enter the short head close from the femur close to its origin and supply blood to it. Also, the superior lateral genicular artery off of the popliteal artery perfuses the muscle distally.

Semitendinosus originates at the ischial tuberosity and inserts on the upper portion of the medial condyle of the tibia. This is a type II muscle. It contains a lengthy tendon and is located posteromedial in the thigh. It shares a tendon with the long head of the bicep femoris at its origin, and it contains an aponeurosis that connects the adjacent surfaces of the two muscles for a distance of about 7.5 cm. The belly of the muscle ends a little below midthigh, which runs on the surface of the semimembranosus as a long, rounded tendon. This tendon curves around the medial condyle of the tibia, and after passing the collateral ligament of the knee it then inserts into the upper part of the tibia medially behind the attachment of the sartorius. It terminates to form the pes anserinus with the sartorius and gracilis. Actions of this muscle are flexion of leg and extension of the thigh. It is innervated the same as the bicep femoris (noted above). Blood supply to this muscle comes mostly from the first perforating branch of the profunda, which is found entering the muscle on its deep lateral surface. Other arteries feed the muscle: the muscular branch of the inferior gluteal artery perfuses the muscle at its origin; the upper portion of the muscle gets fed by the descending branch of MCFA off of the profunda femoral artery; and near the tendon of the muscle distally the inferior medial genicular artery of popliteal artery gives it its blood supply.

Semimembranosus originates at the ischial tuberosity also and inserts at the posterior part of the medial condyle of the tibia. It obtained its name because proximally it is a flattened, wide tendon in the upper thigh. This is a type II and type III muscle that varies in size. It can also be absent. The tendon of this muscle descends and broadens deep to the long head of the bicep femoris and semitendinosus muscle. About midthigh muscle fibers arise from the tendon and converge to a second aponeurosis on the posterior lower part of the muscle. The tendon divides into five parts at the level of the knee, the main one attached to the posterior aspect of the medial condyle of the tibia. The other four components are: series of slips to the medial side of the tibia behind the collateral ligament; deep to the collateral ligament of the tibia, a cord-like tendon to the back part of the medial condyle of the tibia; a thin fascia expansion over the popliteus; and a strong expansion that forms most of the oblique popliteal ligament of the knee joint. The popliteal vessels are overlapped by the muscle, and semimembranosus is overlapped itself by semitendinosus throughout its length. Actions of this muscle are flexion of the leg and extension of the thigh. Blood supply is mostly given by the first perforating branch of the profunda femoral artery, which enters on the deep lateral surface of the muscle. The second or third perforating branch of the profunda also supplies this area of the muscle. The inferior gluteal artery gives blood to the muscle's origin, while a branch of superficial femoral artery gives blood at the insertion of semimembranosus muscle.

A muscular tripod is formed by three muscles: the sartorius, gracilis, and semitendinosus muscle. These three muscles originate and course through three different compartments; each are innervated by different nerves and have different functions, but all share a common insertion site. Each tendon from the three muscles become attached to a flat, broad aponeurosis and is called pes anserinus at the site which they insert on the medial aspect of the tibia.

Anterior Leg Compartment

The leg can be divided into four compartments: anterior, lateral, superficial posterior, and deep posterior. The muscular contents of each compartment will be discussed below (Table 1).

Tibialis anterior is a superficial and easily palpable muscle located lateral to the tibia, which dorsiflexes the foot. Its origin is the lateral condyle and proximal two-thirds of the lateral tibia and the interosseous membrane. It is approximately 25×4 cm^2 and covers the anterior tibial vessels and deep peroneal nerve proximally; then the muscle descends parallel to the tibia ending in a tendon which passes under the superior and inferior retinaculum and crosses the tibia medially at the ankle to insert on the base of the first metatarsal and cuneiform. Insertion variations may include insertion on the talus of the first metatarsal head or proximal hallux phalanx. The tibialis anterior is innervated by the deep peroneal nerve (anterior tibial nerve) from L4 and L5 roots. The tibialis anterior receives its blood supply from direct and recurrent branches of the AT as well as the medial malleolar artery distally in the tendinous portion. As this muscle is key to dorsiflexion, it is not expendable. However, a denervated muscle may be used as a rotational muscle flap for very small defects of the anterior tibia in the middle and lower third of the leg as a superiorly or inferiorly based flap.

EHL is a short, narrow muscle on the anteriolateral aspect of the leg measuring 3×24 cm^2 that extends the hallux and dorsiflexes the foot. Its origin is the middle half of the medial fibula where it is deep to tibialis anterior and EDL. The anterior tibial vessels and deep peroneal nerve lie between EHL and anterior tibialis. As it travels distally it becomes a tendon passing under the superior retinaculum and crossing medially under the inferior retinaculum and inserts into the distal hallux phalanx. In a variation, the tendon unites with EDL and inserts on the second digit. This muscle is also innervated by the deep peroneal nerve and receives direct arterial inflow from the AT as well as medial malleolar artery and dorsalis pedis. It is a type IV Mathes and Nahai classification flap type. Because hallux dorsiflexion is also performed by the extensor hallucis brevis, this is an expendable muscle, but due to its diminutive size it is only useful for distal tibia coverage of small areas by inferior-based pedicle.

(*Text continued on p. 42*)

Table 1 Muscles of the Thigh and Leg

Compartment	Muscle	Origin	Insertion	Action	Innervation	Vascular inflow
The thigh						
Anterior	Tensor fascia lata	ASIS and external lip of iliac crest	Iliotibial tract to lateral condyle of tibia	Abducts and flexes thigh; maintains knee extension; stabilizes knee	Superior gluteal nerve L4,5	Superior and inferior gluteal arteries
	Sartorius	Anterior superior iliac spine	Superiomedial tibia	Flexes thigh; thigh ab-duction/exter-nal rotation	Femoral nerve L2,3	Superficial femoral artery (SFA), genicular arteries
	Quadriceps femoris					
	Rectus femoris	Anterior inferior iliac spine	Base of patella via patella ligament into tibial tuberosity	Extends leg; flexes thigh	Femoral nerve L2,3,4	Profunda femoris directly and descending branch of lateral circumflex femoral artery
	Vastus lateralis	Greater trochanter linea aspera of femur	Base of patella via patella ligament into tibial tuberosity	Extends leg	Femoral nerve L2,3,4	Descending branches of lateral circum-flex femoral artery
	Vastus medialis	Intertrochanteric line and linea aspera of femur	Base of patella via patella ligament into tibial tuberosity	Extends leg	Femoral nerve L2,3,4	SFA; genicular arteries
	Vastus intermedius	Anteriolateral body of femur	Base of patella via patella ligament into tibial tuberosity	Extends leg	Femoral nerve L2,3,4	SFA, profunda fem-oris, descending and transverse branches of lateral circumflex femoral artery

(Continued)

Table 1 Muscles of the Thigh and Leg (*Continued*)

Compartment	Muscle	Origin	Insertion	Action	Innervation	Vascular inflow
	Articularis genus often indistinct from vastus intermedius	Anteriolateral body of femur	Base of patella via patella ligament into tibial tuberosity	Retracts suprapatella bursa proximally in leg extension	Femoral nerve L2,3,4	Femoral artery, profunda femoris, descending and transverse branches of lateral circumflex femoral artery
Medial	Gracilis	Body and inferior ramus of pubis	Superiomedial tibia	Adducts thigh and flexes leg	Obdurator nerve L2,L3	Obdurator artery, medial circumflex femoral artery, SFA and genicular arteries
	Pectineus	Pectin pubis	Pectineal line of femur	Adducts and flexes thigh	Femoral nerve L2,3 nerve branch	Obdurator artery, medial circumflex femoral artery
	Adductor longus	Body of pubis	Linea aspera	Adducts and flexes thigh	Obdurator nerve L2,L3	SFA and first to third profundus perforators, medial circumflex femoral artery
	Adductor brevis	Body and inferior ramus of pubis	Pectineal line of femur	Adducts and flexes thigh	Obdurator nerve L2,L3	SFA and first to third profundus perforators
	Adductor magnus	Inferior ramus of pubis, ischial tuberosity; ramus of ischium	Gluteal tuberosity, linea aspera adductor tubercle of femur	Adducts and extends thigh	Obdurator nerve L2,L3 sciatic nerve L2,3,4	SFA and direct profundus branches
Posterior	Biceps femoris	Long head: ischial tuberosity short head: linea aspera	Fibula head	Extends thigh and flexes leg	Long: tibial division nerve L5 S1 S2 short: common peroneal	Obdurator proximally; profundus perforators distally popliteal and genicular arteries

	Semitendinosus	Ischial tuberosity	Superiomedial tibia	Extends thigh; flexes leg	Tibial division of sciatic nerve L5 S1 S2	Posterior obdurator artery, profundus branches popliteal and genicular artery
	Semimembranosus	Ischial tuberosity	Posteriomedial tibia condyle	Extends thigh; flexes leg	Tibial division of sciatic nerve L5 S1 S2	Posterior obdurator artery, profundus branches popliteal and genicular artery
The leg						
Anterior	Tibialis anterior	Superior half of lateral tibia and lateral condyle	Base first metatarsal inferior and medial cuneiform; variations may insert on hallux or talus	Dorsiflex foot; inverts foot	Deep peroneal nerve L4 and L5	Direct branches from anterior tibial artery and anterior tibial recurrent artery: tendon supplied by anterior medial malleolar artery and dorsalis pedis
	Extensor hallucis longus	Mid-medial fibula	Becomes a tendon and passes mediallsdorsal aspect base phalanx: sometimes with EDL	Extends hallux dorsiflex foot	Deep peroneal nerve L5 and S1	Direct branches from anterior tibial artery and anterior medial malleolar artery and dorsalis pedis; sometimes peroneal artery perforators

(*Continued*)

Table 1 Muscles of the Thigh and Leg *(Continued)*

Compartment	Muscle	Origin	Insertion	Action	Innervation	Vascular inflow
	Extensor digitorum longus	Anterior surface superior two-thirds fibula interosseous membrane and lateral tibia condyle	Middle and distal phalanx of lateral four digits	Extends lateral 4 toes; dorsiflexes foot	Deep peroneal nerve L5 and S1	Direct anterior tibial artery branches and anterior lateral malleolar artery branches and dorsalis pedis
	Peroneus tertius sometimes absent	Described as fifth slip of EDL medial inferior fibula origin	Medial dorsal fifth metatarsal	Eversion and dorsiflex; on foot	Deep peroneal nerve L5 and S1	Direct branches from anterior tibial artery anterior lateral malleolar antery
Lateral	Peroneus longus (more superficial than brevis)	Lateral proximal two-thirds of fibula lateral condyle (tendon changes direction below lateral malleolus and on cuboid	By two slips attatches to lateral base of first metatarsal and medial cuneiform; variation: insert base of second metatarsal	Plantarflexes; foot eversion	Superficial peroneal S1 and S2	Proximal: inferior lateral geniculate aretery main belly and tendon: peroneal artery and perforators joining anterior lateral malleolar
	Peroneus brevis	Lateral distal two-thirds fibula sometimes fuses with longus	Dorsal lateral base of fifth metatarsal	Plantarflexes; foot eversion	Superficial peroneal nerve L5 S1 S2	Peroneal artery and perforators joining anterior lateral malleolar artery
Superficial posterior	Gastrocnemius	Lateral head from lateral condyle; medial head from popliteal surface of femur	Posterior surface of calcaneus	Flexes knee, plantarflexes; raises heel while walking; force and propulsion	Tibial nerve S1 and surface of muscle	Medial and lateral sural artery from popliteal a. medial and lateral artery and anterior and posterior medial and lateral malleolar a to Achilles tendon.

	Soleus	Posterior head of fibula and mid posterior tibia	Posterior calcaneoues Achilles tendon	Plantarflexion; stabilizes leg and foot when standing	Posterior tibial nerve S1 and S2	Muscular branches of popliteal a, posterior tibial
	Plantaris	Lower lateral supracondylar line	Tendon divides gastrocnemius and soleus then fuses to become Achilles tendon	Sometimes absent; plantarflexion; knee extension	Tibial nerve S1 and S2	Sural and malleolar arteries
Deep posterior	Popliteus	Lateral surface of the lateral condyle and lateral meniscus	Posterior tibia superior to the soleal line	Flexes knee; unlocks knee by rotating tibia midially on femur	Tibial nerve L4, L5, S1	Directly from popliteal arteries and sural arteries and lateral genicular arteries and posterior tibial recurrent artery
	Flexor hallucis longus	Distal two-thirds posterior fibula	Base of distal phalanx of hallux	Flexes hallux; plantarflexion	Posterior tibial nerve S2 and S3	Branches from peroneal and posterior tibial artery
	Flexor digitorum longus	Posteriomedial tibia inferior to soleal line	Base of disal phalanx lateral 4 digits	Plantarflexion; flexes lateral 4 digits	Tibial nerve L5, S1, S2	Branches from posterior tibial and peroneal artery
	Tibialis posterior	Posteriolateral tibia, interosseous membrane, superiomedial fibula	Navicular, cuneiform, cuboid, and base 2,3,4 metatarsals	Inverts foot; plantarflexion	Posterior tibial nerve L4 and L5	Posterior tibial a and peroneal artery

Abbreviation: ASIS; anterior superior iliac spine.

EDL is a pennant 4 × 35 cm^2 long, thin muscle on the anterolateral aspect of the leg lateral to tibialis anterior originating from the lateral condyle of the tibia and proximal three-fourths of the medial fibula and the interosseous membrane. Proximally this muscle lies lateral to the AT and deep peroneal nerve. EDL becomes tendinous in the midleg and continues distally to pass under the superior retinaculum. As it passes under the inferior retinaculum, it splits into four slips to insert on the middle and distal phalanges of the second through fifth digits. There may be accessory slips to the hallux in variants. This is a type IV muscle supplied by the AT directly and the medial malleolar artery and is innervated by the deep peroneal nerve. EDL serves to extend the toes and dorsiflex the foot. Extensor digitorum brevis (EDB) will preserve the extension at the metacarpal phalangeal joint (MP) but distal interphalngeal joint (DIP) extension will be lost if this muscle is sacrificed; therefore it is usually transferred in a function preserving manner as a superiorly based flap to cover very small distal third tibia defects.

Lateral Leg Compartment

The peroneus longus can evert and plantarflex the foot as well as support the arches of the foot. PL originates from the head and upper two-thirds of the lateral fibula. It is 4 × 10 cm^2 between the gap of its insertion and the head and the shaft of the fibula the common peroneal nerve passes. The muscle is short and ends in a long tendon, which travels posterior to the lateral malleolus into a groove it shares with PB. It crosses the calcaneous obliquely on the lateral surface and then traverses obliquely across the undersurface of the foot to insert on the lateral side of the base of the first metatarsal and cuneiform. This is a type II muscle innervated by the superficial peroneal nerve and supplied by muscular branches of the peroneal and to a lesser degree the AT. This flap based superiorly can be used to cover small middle third defects or can be included in a fibula flap.

PB flexes and everts the foot and is expendable if PL is intact. It originates from the lower third of the lateral fibula. The superficial peroneal nerve motor branches enter the PB proximally while the sensory nerve travels superficially on the belly of the muscle deep to the crural fascia. The PB is 15 × 3 cm^2 and is a type II muscle. It ends in a tendon that passes behind the lateral malleolus anterior to PL. The tendon continues under the retinaculum lateral to the calcaneous to insert on the base of the fifth metatarsal. It is vascularized from direct peroneal branches and perforating branches joining the lateral malleolar artery. It can be raised as a flap based on the proximal dominant pedicle and may reach upper lower third small defects.

Superficial Posterior Leg Compartment

The gastrocnemius muscle provides force and propulsion in running, jumping, and walking. Along with the soleus it is the chief plantar flexor of the foot. The gastrocnemius is also a knee flexor. It is a 20 × 8 cm^2 muscle that is type I. It originates on the medial condyle of the femur and the lateral head of the femoral condyle (which often contains a sesamoid bone in the tendinous origin of the head) where it forms the inferior medial and lateral border of the popliteal fossa. The medial head is larger and descends more distally than the lateral head. The fleshy muscle descends until midcalf where it inserts into a broad aponeurosis and inserts into the calcaneous via the tendon calcaneous. The plantaris muscle can be identified in most individuals separating the gastrocnemius and soleus muscles. It is innervated by the tibial nerve and is vascularized by the sural arteries. The skin over the medial gastrocnemius receives sensory innervations from the saphenous nerve, and laterally the sural nerve innervates the skin over the lateral gastrocnemius. Either or both heads of the gastrocnemius are expendable if the soleus is intact. The gastrocnemius based superiorly is used to cover the knee and upper third tibia defects. Distally based flap can be used to cover middle third leg defects.

The soleus muscle is a large bipenniform muscle deep to the gastrocnemius that is 8×28 cm^2 and originates medially on the middle medial third of the tibia and laterally on the posterior fibula head and body. The soleus steadies the foot while standing and has more fatigue-resistant fibers than the gastrocnemius muscle, but it also plantarflexes. It is a type II muscle innervated by the posterior tibial and medial popliteal nerves. It is supplied by the popliteal artery and posterior tibial and peroneal arteries. It inserts similarly to the gastrocnemius muscle to the calcaneous by the Achilles tendon. It is longer than the gastrocnemius and is a work-horse for middle and even upper lower third leg defects.

Deep Posterior Leg Compartment

FHL originates from the distal two-thirds of the posterior fibula, the interosseous membrane, and the intermuscular septum. It is 3×20 cm^2 and gradually tapers to a tendon that grooves the lower posterior tibia and talus. It inserts on the base of the distal hallux phalanx. FHL is innervated by the posterior tibial nerve and supplied by the peroneal artery and is a type IV muscle. This is an uncommonly used flap that can cover very small lower third defects. FHL acts as a weak plantar flexor.

FDL is medial to FHL and flexes the terminal phalanx of the second through fifth digits. FDL can be sacrificed if flexor digitorum brevis (FDB) is intact. FDL originates from the body of the tibia on the posterior surface just below the soleal line. The muscle ends in a tendon that traverses nearly the entire posterior surface of the muscle. It crosses the tibialis posterior and passes behind the medial malleolus accompanied by the tibialis posterior but separated from it by a fibrous septum. It passes deep to the flexor retinaculum and enters the sole of the foot and inserts on the base of the distal phalanx of the second through fifth toes. The FDL is innervated by the tibial nerve and is supplied by the PT. It is an uncommonly used flap but can be used to cover small lower third defects.

NAMED ANATOMIC SPACES

Femoral Triangle

The femoral triangle is bound superiorly by the inguinal ligament, laterally by the sartorius, and medially by the adductor longus. The floor of the triangle is muscular, involving the pectineus, iliopsoas, and adductor longus. Its contents include the femoral vessels, lymphatics, and femoral nerve. The vessels without the nerve are encircled in the femoral sheath which is an extension of abdominal fascia (transversalis and iliacus).

Adductor Canal

The adductor canal is bounded posteriomedially by the adductor longus and magnus, laterally by the vastus medialis, and anteriorly by the sartorius. The contents include the superficial femoral vessels with the vein taking a posterior position. As the vessels exit the adductor hiatus through a tendinous opening in the adductor magnus, they enter the popliteal fossa, and they take on the name popliteal artery and vein.

Popliteal Fossa

The popliteal fossa is a diamond-shaped region posterior to the knee roofed by skin and subcutaneous tissue, bounded by semitendinosus/semimembranosus and biceps femoris and the heads of the gastrocnemius inferiorly. The contents include a fat pad, the bursa, lymphatics, the popliteal vessels, tibial and common peroneal nerve, and the lesser saphenous vein and posterior femoral cutaneous nerve in the superficial fascia. Within the popliteal fossa, the geniculate branches branch and are named lateral and medial, superior middle, and inferior genicular arteries.

REFERENCE

1. Moore KL. Clinically Oriented Anatomy. 2nd ed. Baltimore: Williams and Wilkins, 1985: 432.

3

Orthopedic Treatment of the Traumatized Lower Extremity

Steven P. Kalandiak
Department of Orthopedics and Rehabilitation, Miller School of Medicine, University of Miami, Miami, Florida, U.S.A.

INTRODUCTION

The severely traumatized lower extremity presents a complex problem that often requires the skills of surgeons familiar with orthopedic, soft tissue, and microvascular techniques. Although this combination of skills occasionally exists in the hands of a single "orthoplastic" surgeon, it is far more common for a team of orthopedic, plastic, and vascular surgeons to share responsibility for these devastating injuries. This chapter provides an overview of the orthopedic management of the severely traumatized lower extremity and discusses the role of the orthopedist in the team approach to these injuries. It begins with a section on evaluation and management, then discusses special problems facing the surgeon treating the severely traumatized limb, and concludes by discussing techniques of fixation and reconstruction.

INITIAL EVALUATION AND MANAGEMENT

When a severely compromised limb presents to the emergency department, immediate involvement of the orthopedic and, when necessary, vascular, and/or plastic services optimizes patient care. Although the initial trauma resuscitation assumes primary importance, with proper teamwork the initial care of the injured leg can often be carried out nearly simultaneously. The orthopedist's initial role is the immediate evaluation and stabilization of the injured extremity to prevent additional local and systemic injury. Obvious dislocations and displaced fracture fragments causing pressure or tension on skin, soft tissues, and neurovascular structures should be reduced or realigned promptly. The size of open wounds and severity of soft-tissue injuries are assessed, and the limb evaluated for vascular compromise and compartment syndrome. Open wounds are then sterilely dressed, and the limb is temporarily stabilized with a combination of splintage, traction, and occasional external fixation.

Open wounds and soft-tissue injury grades are provisionally assigned according to the classification system of Gustilo (1,2). Patients with minor open wounds should receive a first-generation cephalosporin, with the addition of an aminoglycoside for severe open wounds. In cases of soil or farm contamination, or severe crush, a penicillin derivative is added to provide anaerobic (clostridial) coverage. All open fracture patients should also receive appropriate tetanus prophylaxis.

Vascular status of the limb is then assessed by evaluating palpable pulses and performing Doppler exam and ankle-brachial indices if there is a potential vascular injury. If vascular injury is present, the decision whether to perform formal angiography in the radiology suite or a one-shot angiogram in the operating room or to proceed with immediate surgical exploration must be individualized according to the condition of the patient and the limb.

The awake patient should be examined for the signs of compartment syndrome, but in the polytrauma patient, sedation, loss of consciousness, and distracting injury make clinical evaluation difficult. If there is a question of compartment syndrome and the patient is not able to participate in the exam, measurement of compartment pressures becomes crucial. Even when blood flow appears adequate, careful continued monitoring is necessary as vascular occlusion or compartment syndrome may develop in a delayed fashion in association with intimal vessel injury or resuscitation and reperfusion of an injured extremity.

Once the initial stabilization and evaluation have occurred, the orthopedist must determine whether an operative emergency exists. Open fractures, mangled and/or dysvascular extremities, compartment syndrome, and traumatic amputations all present threats to limb that should receive operative care within the first few hours after injury, unless threats to life itself supervene. Irreducible dislocations, hip dislocation, and femoral neck fracture (in the young patient) are also considered operative emergencies. Fractures of the femoral shaft, while not truly limb-threatening emergencies, present physiologic challenges and difficulties of immobilization not seen in fractures at the knee and below. Early fixation of the femoral shaft, either by intramedullary or by external fixation, contributes to both the resuscitation of the limb and of the overall patient. A grossly unstable pelvis, while not truly an extremity injury, may represent the only immediately life-threatening orthopedic injury, and its stabilization should thus receive appropriate priority.

Although full radiographic evaluation should be deferred until the critical patient is stabilized, single-spot radiographs of the injured extremities, obtained as soon as practical after the usual c-spine, chest, and pelvis films, are often useful in forming a complete picture of the patient's injuries. However, when truly life-threatening injuries are present and require immediate operative attention, injured limbs should be quickly and provisionally stabilized, and X-ray evaluation deferred to a later time. If complete radiographs can be obtained in a timely fashion, they are of course beneficial, but in emergent cases, if the patient and the operating room are ready, it is often faster and more efficient to bring the patient to the room and complete the radiographic evaluation there rather than wait for films to be obtained in the emergency department.

CLASSIFICATION OF OPEN FRACTURES AND SEVERE SOFT TISSUE INJURY

By far, the most common operative emergency the orthopedist will see in the setting of lower extremity trauma is an open fracture. In 1976, Gustilo and Anderson (1) reviewed over a thousand open fractures of long bones and proposed the following classification: type I—open fracture with a clean wound less than 1 cm long, type II—open fracture with a laceration longer than 1 cm without extensive soft-tissue damage, and type III—open fracture with high energy of injury and severe soft-tissue damage. In 1984, Gustilo et al. (2) further subdivided type III fractures as: type IIIA—adequate soft-tissue coverage despite extensive soft-tissue laceration or flaps, or high-energy trauma irrespective of the size of the wound; type IIIB—extensive soft-tissue injury loss with periosteal stripping and bone exposure. This is usually associated with massive contamination and is generally taken to mean that rotational or free flap coverage is required; and type IIIC—open fracture associated with arterial injury requiring repair.

Although the initial work of Gustilo and Anderson (1), and interpretation of it, placed significant emphasis on the size of the wound, their subsequent work (2) emphasized the degree of contamination and soft-tissue injury. Subsequent authors (3,4) have emphasized the degree of soft-tissue injury to an even greater degree, adding extensive contamination, close-range shotgun, and high-velocity gunshot wounds, displaced segmental fractures, fractures with diaphyseal loss, vascular injury requiring repair, any barnyard wound, crush from a fast-moving vehicle, and associated compartment syndrome to the list of factors that mandate a type III classification, regardless of the size of the skin wound. Their classification is prognostic: with modern fracture care techniques, the infection rate in type I open fractures should approach that of closed injuries, the rate for type II and IIIA up to 7%, and the rates for types IIIB from 10% to 50%, and IIIC from 25% to 50% (4).

An alternative classification system, utilized more frequently in the European literature, is that of Tscherne, which uses similar grades of I, II, and III according to wound size, contamination, and fracture pattern, and adds a grade IV for incomplete and complete amputations (5). In addition, Tscherne has given an important classification system for the severity of soft-tissue injury in closed fractures (5) as: grade 0—indirect force and negligible soft-tissue damage; grade

I—low-to-moderate energy, with superficial abrasion or contusion of the overlying soft tissue; grade II—resulting from direct, violent force, with severe fracture pattern and deep contaminated abrasions and/or significant muscle contusion, and putting the extremity at risk for compartment syndrome; and grade III—extensive crush with subcutaneous "degloving" and arterial injury or established compartment syndrome.

OPEN FRACTURES—TREATMENT

When an open wound accompanies a fracture, operative irrigation and debridement should be carried out as promptly as possible. If the patient's condition or the available resources prohibit a trip to the operating room within a few hours time, removal of superficial gross contamination and provisional irrigation of already exposed surfaces may be carried out in the emergency department, but the wound should not be explored and the depths of the wound should not be exposed, as the emergency room environment lacks sterility and exposure of the deep wound may destabilize clot and increase bleeding. A sterile dressing should then be placed on the wound, left in place until the definitive debridement, and the limb immobilized in the appropriate fashion.

Once the patient stabilizes, additional care of the extremity should occur in the operating room. Ideally this should occur within a few hours of injury. After standard sterile preparation of the extremity, the surgeon should meticulously irrigate and debride any open wounds, removing all contaminants and any devitalized skin, subcutaneous tissue, muscle, and devitalized extra-articular bone. Although the majority of the case should be done without one, a tourniquet should be placed prior to starting the procedure and inflated if necessary to control arterial bleeding or to improve visualization, particularly when dissecting neurovascular structures.

In the past, cultures were often taken pre- and postdebridement in order to determine antibiotic therapy. However, Lee (6) retrospectively reviewed 245 open fractures and found that only 8% of organisms grown on predebridement cultures eventually caused infection. In addition, of cases that did become infected, predebridement cultures grew the infecting organism only 22% and postdebridement cultures only 42% of the time. Because the predictive value of routinely culturing open wounds is so low, most have abandoned it, performing cultures only in those situations where infection is present.

We typically begin with a preliminary irrigation to remove gross contaminants and clot to better visualize the anatomic structures of the limb. Debridement is then carried out, interspersed with irrigation as necessary to remove debris and improve visualization. At the conclusion of the debridement, several additional liters of pulsatile lavage are utilized, for a total ranging from 4 L for relatively clean to a total of 12–16 L for large, grossly contaminated wounds. High-pressure pulsatile lavage is a useful adjunct to the debridement, providing efficient cleansing of contaminants from some bone surfaces and the soft tissues; however, high-pressure lavage should not be used on neurovascular structures, and may impel contaminants further into the bone and cause damage to bone structure and osteocytes at the fracture site. Antibiotics added to the irrigant may kill bacteria, but are also potentially toxic to host cells. Bhandari et al. (7–9) and Dirschl et al. (10,11) have produced numerous studies on the effect of pulsatile lavage on bacterial contamination, osteocytes function, and fracture healing. Anglen (12) has recently provided an excellent review of wound irrigation in musculoskeletal injury. Although evidence is mixed, on balance pulsatile lavage seems to be beneficial.

Approach to debridement should be systematic, so that no area of the wound is neglected. Beginning at the surface, one should sharply excise contused or contaminated skin a millimeter or two into healthy tissue in areas where the skin is plentiful. In areas such as the foot or front of the tibia, where skin coverage is more tenuous, it may be better to retain skin that has not declared itself and reexamine it at a later time.

At the time of injury, fractured segments of bone may protrude far beyond the wound and then recoil back into the limb, carrying contaminants with them. In addition, when injuries have a crush component, the zone of compromised soft tissue may extend well beyond the wound—indeed at times no wound may be present. In these cases, it is critically important that the skin wound be extended longitudinally and that the fascia of all affected compartments be opened until the entire zone of injury and contamination has been visualized so that all contaminated and devitalized tissues may be debrided. If there is a suspicion of compartment syndrome, the entire compartment should be opened. Only by extending the incision until normal tissues have been reached can one be assured of an adequate debridement.

In the setting of high-energy trauma, the size of the skin wound may often belie the underlying soft-tissue injury. Figures 1 and 2 show an open tibial shaft fracture. The limb was provisionally aligned with a half pin external fixator. The traumatic wound is the transverse laceration above the ankle. The wound was extended longitudinally to expose internal degloving that extended more than halfway up the leg toward the knee. Figures 3 and 4 show the true extent of the underlying injury.

The next layers of debridement are the muscle compartments themselves, with their accompanying nerves, vessels, and tendons. Contaminated and devitalized muscle provides the major substrate for bacterial infection and must be scrupulously removed. However, muscle viability is often difficult to judge and the surgeon may face a decision on whether to retain or discard muscle of uncertain quality. Scully et al. (13) have listed four factors: color, contractility, consistency, and capacity to bleed to allow the surgeon to judge the viability of the muscle and debride appropriately. Because any one parameter may be misleading, it is important to consider the combination of these factors as well as the degree of injury when debriding muscle. If the area of muscle loss is small compared to the whole compartment, debridement may quickly extend back to healthy muscle, but when an entire compartment is threatened, significant functional gains may result if even a small portion of its contents is maintained. In this situation, questionable muscle may be

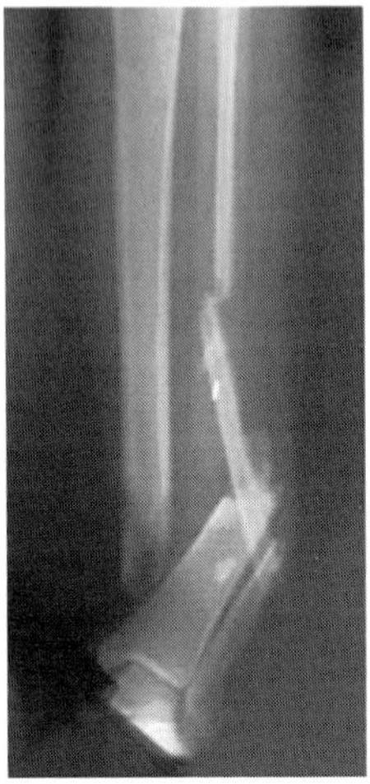

Figure 1 X ray of a high energy open tibial shaff fracture.

left and reevaluated in the operating room within one to two days so that it will have time to declare its viability.

Nerves and vessels should be dissected carefully and preserved. Reparable nerve injuries should be fixed prior to closure, although the prognosis with tibial nerve injury is particularly poor. Vessels requiring repair should be addressed rapidly, as the likelihood of limb salvage drops dramatically as warm ischemia time moves beyond six to eight hours. If a limb is judged dysvascular but salvageable, the initial debridement and stabilization should be provisional and rapid, so that blood flow may be restored as quickly as possible. At times, a temporary shunt can rapidly restore blood flow and allow

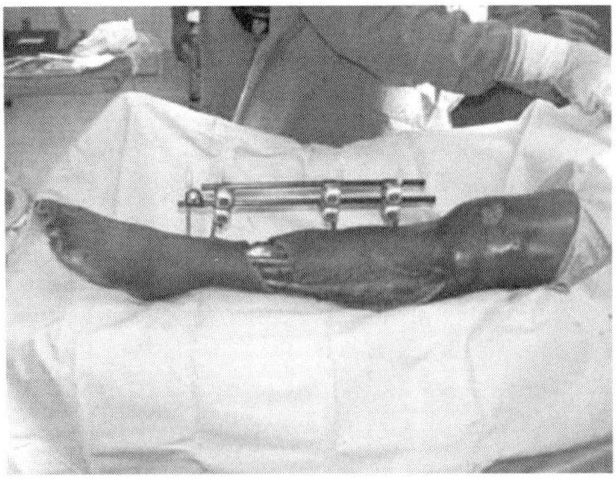

Figure 2 Temporary half pin external fixation of the limb shown above. The distal transverse wound is from the trauma. The proximal longitudinal incision was made to expose the internal degloving.

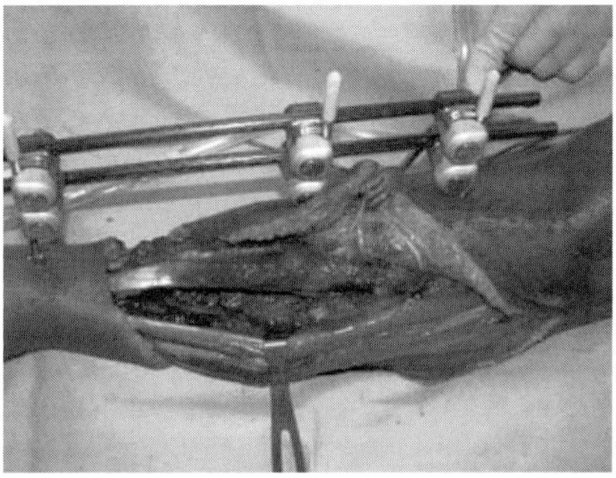

Figure 3 The extent of internal degloving.

a more thorough and definitive debridement and stabilization before the final vascular repair.

Debridement of the bone itself completes this phase of the operation. Diaphyseal bone that has been completely stripped of its blood supply should be discarded in almost all cases. Surfaces remaining in the wound should be mechanically cleansed and irrigated. Avascular segments of the articular surface require greater judgment. Their debridement is permissible if they are grossly contaminated or obviously nonreconstructible, but, in general, the decision as to whether or not to discard portions of the joint surface is a sophisticated one and should be left to the surgeon who will be performing the definitive reconstruction. Additional pulsatile lavage completes this phase of fracture care. At this point, the fracture may be either provisionally or definitively stabilized, depending on patient condition, surgeon capability, and available resources.

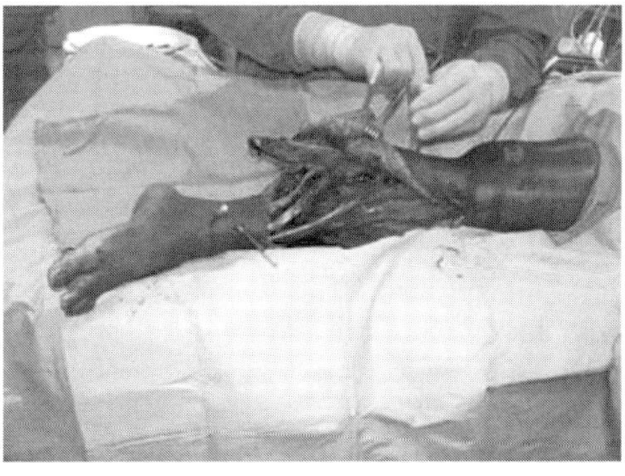

Figure 4 The "true" injury. Aside from incising the skin and opening the compartment, no additional dissection was performed.

COMPARTMENT SYNDROME

Increased pressure within an enclosed fascial compartment, if unrecognized, may result in swelling and muscle ischemia, followed by contractures and irreversible injury to muscle, nerve, and function of the limb. First recognized by Volkmann (14) in 1881, compartment syndrome has received increased attention in recent years as our awareness of this entity has grown. Simply put, increased pressure within an enclosed space decreases capillary blood flow below the level necessary to provide tissue viability. This increased pressure may result from either an increased volume in the space, e.g., from bleeding, or from a decrease in the size of the space, such as from an excessively tight cast. In the setting of lower extremity trauma, fracture, soft tissue, and arterial injury, as well as burns, reperfusion injury, and tight circumferential cast and dressings may be the cause. As pressure within the compartment rises, the decreased capillary flow results in shunting of flow through, rather than into the compartment. If this continues, ischemia of the muscles produces tissue necrosis, which in turn produces fluid and electrolyte shifts that further compound the problem. If the syndrome continues unrecognized, the muscles die and contract, resulting in severe and permanent disability. In severe cases, the resulting rhabdomyolysis may result in acute renal failure.

Of vital importance in arriving at a prompt and correct diagnosis of compartment syndrome is a high index of suspicion. Although the five P's, pulselessness, pallor, paresthesia, paralysis, and pain with passive stretch, have classically been listed as the signs of compartment syndrome, the first four are, in fact, signs of a compartment syndrome that is already quite advanced. Only pain, often out of proportion to what is expected for the injury, and exacerbated by passive stretch of the muscles in the compartment, provides a sensitive clinical indicator of a developing compartment syndrome. In the unconscious or head-injured patient, these signs are obviously highly unreliable and the index of suspicion becomes critically important. If clinical signs of compartment syndrome are clear, the surgeon should proceed to fasciotomy emergently.

When clinical signs are equivocal or the patient cannot be examined because of mental status, measurement of compartment pressures is indicated. The most common technique in clinical practice involves the use of the Stryker Stic system with a side-port needle to measure intracompartmental pressure. The device is small, portable, relatively inexpensive, and easy to use. The other common technique is the Whiteside's technique, which uses a three-way stopcock, i.v. tubing, and a manometer or pressure transducer to measure intracompartmental pressure. Techniques using special wick and slit catheters have also been described but are less common. In the operating room or intensive care unit, where an a-line setup is available, it is sometimes used to measure the compartment pressure directly, but the efficacy of this technique is unproven. One additional consideration that further emphasizes the importance of clinical evaluation is that Moed and Thorderson (15) have shown that techniques using a simple needle may read an average of 18–19 mm higher than a side-port or slit needle.

The exact pressure measurement at which compartments should be released is still somewhat controversial. Mubarak et al. (16) and Matsen et al. (17) advocated release when the pressures reached 30–40 and 45 mmHg, respectively. More recently, the role of blood pressure in providing compartment perfusion has drawn attention. McQueen and Court-Brown (18) recommended considering fasciotomy when the difference between compartment and diastolic pressure was less than 30 mmHg, and Heppenstal et al. (19) advocated fasciotomy when the difference between compartment pressure and mean arterial pressure (delta P) was less than 40 mmHg. Thus, one may see that periods of prolonged hypotension, which lower the diastolic and mean arterial pressures, increase the risk of compartment syndrome considerably.

In cases where clinical examination is available, it always plays an extremely important role. The consequence of failing to release a compartment syndrome is so great that fasciotomy should generally be performed on the basis of clinical signs and symptoms, with pressure measurements reserved for cases which are unclear and for head injured patients. The presence of an open wound should not be taken to imply that compartments have been released. In fact, compartment syndrome frequently accompanies open fracture when the soft-tissue injury is severe.

When clinical signs of compartment syndrome are present, any circumferential cast or dressing, including the padding under a cast, should be completely released. In a head-injured patient, casts and circumferential dressings should be avoided whenever possible. If clinical signs of compartment syndrome persist after release of any circumferential wrapping, the patient should go to the operating room for fasciotomy. In the thigh and leg, the clinical picture is usually fairly clear, but in the foot both clinical diagnosis and pressure measurement are more difficult, and index of suspicion becomes even more important. Again, if the diagnosis is equivocal, it is better to err on the side of performing the fasciotomy rather than waiting and missing the chance to avert a potentially disastrous outcome.

Techniques of Fasciotomy

Thigh—Although less common than compartment syndrome of the leg and foot, thigh compartment syndrome can occur usually in association with femur fracture or a direct crushing injury. There are three compartments in the thigh—anterior (quadriceps), posterior (hamstrings), and medial (adductors). Because the majority of the femoral shaft is cloaked by the quadriceps, with the posterior and medial compartments having virtually only tendinous attachments to the shaft, an anterior compartment release through a straight lateral incision is usually sufficient to release a thigh compartment syndrome. If the posterior compartment needs release, it can be accessed from the lateral incision through the lateral intermuscular septum. The adductor compartment can be released through a separate medial incision if necessary.

Leg—The most common compartment syndrome encountered in the lower extremity occurs in the leg. The leg contains four compartments: anterior, lateral, superficial posterior, and deep posterior, all of which must be released. Two basic techniques exist: the first, the perifibular approach, popularized by Matsen et al. (17) utilizes a single lateral incision to release all four compartments. The second, a two-incision technique, uses an anterolateral incision for the anterior and lateral compartments and a posteromedial incision for the two posterior compartments.

To perform a single-incision fasciotomy, the skin is incised laterally, over the fibula from its head to the ankle. The anterior and lateral compartments are identified and their fascia incised the entire length of the compartments, just anterior and posterior to their intermuscular septum. A lateral release of the superficial posterior compartment follows. Finally, the interval between the lateral and superficial posterior compartments is developed and the deep posterior compartment opened just behind the fibula. The peroneal nerve divides as it wraps around the fibular neck, with the superficial peroneal branch running just below the fascia of the lateral compartment and then piercing the fascia several centimeters above the ankle and the deep peroneal traversing the interosseous membrane from lateral to medial on the floor of the anterior compartment. These must be protected, particularly in trauma, when the anatomy is distorted.

Double-incision fasciotomy is performed through two incisions that are approximately opposite each other on the leg. The first is anterolateral, centered over the septum between the anterior and lateral compartments. These compartments are opened a centimeter in front of and behind the septum from the level of muscle origin proximally extending down to below the level of the musculotendinous junctions.

A second posteromedial incision is then created a centimeter or two behind the tibia. The saphenous nerve and vein are identified and protected. The fascia overlying the gastroc-soleus complex is easily identified and released. Distally, the deep posterior compartment is easily seen, but proximally, the soleus origin must be reflected back off the tibia to identify and release the deep posterior compartment.

Foot—classically, the description of the foot included four compartments—medial, central, lateral, and interosseous. More recently, Manoli and Weber (20) have identified nine—medial (abductor hallucis and flexor hallucis brevis), superficial (flexor digitorum brevis, flexor digitorum longus tendons, and lumbricals), lateral (abductor digiti minimi and flexor digiti minimi brevis), adductor (adductor hallucis), calcaneal (quadratus plantae), and the four interosseous compartments, and recommended a variation on former methods of foot fasciotomy.

Their recommended technique requires a 6-cm medial incision starting just anterior to the abductor hallucis origin and paralleling the heel pad. The medial compartment is opened longitudinally, leaving a strip of fascia below the abductor. The abductor is retracted superiorly and the far wall of the compartment is incised to open the calcaneal compartment. This should be done with great care because the lateral plantar nerve lies immediately behind that fascial plane. Proceeding below the fascia of the medial compartment leads to the superficial and through it to the lateral compartment. Once this has been accomplished, two dorsal incisions are made, over the second and fourth metatarsals. The four interosseous spaces are released and then the first dorsal and plantar interossei are retracted off the medial side of the second metatarsal to reveal the roof of the adductor compartment, which is also released.

THE MANGLED EXTREMITY

One of the most difficult decisions any orthopedist must face is whether to attempt salvage of a mangled extremity or perform amputation. Sometimes trauma to the limb is so extensive that even with an intact vascular supply, the prognosis for successful salvage is poor. However, the relative rarity of injury this severe, the unique condition of each severely traumatized limb, and the lack of prospective comparative data on salvage versus amputation make decision making difficult. In addition, outside major trauma centers, very few surgeons have a significant experience with these injuries. Although loss of limb is traumatic for the patient, futile attempts at salvaging the unsalvageable can cause a protracted course of multiple surgeries, prolonged hospitalizations, and dramatically increased health-care costs while ultimately resulting in function that is worse than the patient would have obtained from immediate amputation.

As the mangled extremity has received greater attention, trauma surgeons have recognized a need to develop a system of identifying those extremities that would do poorly with attempted salvage, either by identifying characteristics of injury which have a poor prognosis or by developing scoring systems that allow the surgeon to determine which extremities are not salvageable.

Lange et al. (21) retrospectively reviewed 23 open, high-energy tibial fractures with limb-threatening vascular compromise. Based on their data, they considered complete anatomic disruption of the tibial nerve and crush injury with warm ischemia time greater than six hours to be absolute indications for primary amputation. Serious associated trauma, severe ipsilateral foot trauma, and an anticipated protracted course to obtain soft-tissue coverage and tibial reconstitution were considered to be relative indications.

Caudle and Stern (22) reported their results in caring for 62 type III open tibial shaft fractures. Eleven type IIIA fractures resulted in three nonunions, no deep infections, and no secondary amputations. Of 42 type IIIB fractures, 15 progressed to nonunion, 12 to deep infection, and seven to secondary amputation. When the 24 IIIB fractures that underwent flap coverage less than one week after injury were considered, results improved to five nonunions, two deep infections, and two secondary amputations. Of nine type IIIC fractures, seven ultimately had amputations and the two who did not had poor results. Based on this, they concluded that the severity of the initial injury was the most important factor in determining prognosis. They concurred with Lange's absolute indications for primary amputation and added a plea for strong consideration for primary amputation for type IIIC injuries with a severe soft-tissue injury component. When limbs were considered potentially salvageable, they advocated soft-tissue coverage within a week to decrease the risk of infection, nonunion, and amputation.

The past decade has seen the creation of a number of scoring systems designed to discriminate salvageable from unsalvageable limbs based on data available early in the evaluation of patients with severe skeletal and soft-tissue injuries. Most often used to date has been the Mangled Extremity Severity Score (MESS). In two separate reports in 1990, Helfet et al. (23) and Johansen et al. (24) reported on the MESS, a new scale that they found to be highly predictive of the need for amputation. Patients received a score based on energy of injury, degree of shock, length of time and degree of ischemia, and age. The MESS was developed by retrospectively reviewing the data on 26 severely injured extremities and then prospectively applying it to an additional 26 severely injured limbs. In both the retrospective and the prospective series, the MESS functioned flawlessly, predicting both need for amputation and the possibility of salvage with 100% sensitivity and specificity. Subsequent studies have been less accurate.

Robertson (25) reviewed 152 patients with severely injured lower limbs and retrospectively applied the MESS to their admissions data to see if it accurately predicted their outcome. He found that the score was highly successful in predicting the need for immediate amputation, correctly identifying 25 of 30. However, it was much less successful at identifying those patients who subsequently underwent delayed amputation, correctly predicting only 16 of 65. All patients who avoided amputation were correctly identified.

Durham et al. (26) used the MESS and three other scoring systems to retrospectively review a decade of severe extremity trauma at their institution and found that while all of the scoring systems were able to identify the majority of patients who required amputation, none were able to predict functional outcome, and prediction in individual patients was problematic. Furthermore, Bonanni et al. (27) found that attempting to use these same four indices to avoid prolonged reconstructive efforts was futile.

Recently, Bosse et al. (28) as part of a large, prospective multicenter study on severely traumatized limbs, reviewed 556 high-energy, lower-extremity injuries using five injury-severity scoring systems designed to assist in the decision-making process. The analysis did not validate the clinical utility of any of the lower-extremity injury-severity scores. Low scores could be used to predict limb-salvage potential. However, the converse was not true. They concluded that lower-extremity injury-severity scores at or above the amputation threshold should be used cautiously by a surgeon who must decide the fate of a lower extremity with a high-energy injury.

Georgiadis et al. (29) compared the long-term outcomes and the quality of life in patients who had an open fracture of the tibial shaft with severe soft-tissue loss managed with either limb salvage with a free flap or with early below-the-knee amputation. The patients who had limb salvage had more complications, more operative procedures, and a longer stay in the hospital than the patients who had an early amputation. The long-term functional results for 16 patients who had a successful limb-salvage procedure were compared with those for 18 patients who had a below-the-knee amputation. The patients who had had a successful limb-salvage procedure took significantly more time to achieve full weight bearing, were less willing or able to work, and had higher hospital charges than the patients managed with early amputation, and significantly more patients who had limb salvage considered themselves severely disabled.

In contrast, Hertel et al. (30) retrospectively reviewed 18 patients with traumatic lower leg amputation compared to 21 who underwent complex microvascular reconstruction. Although they also found a greater number of interventions and rehabilitation time for the reconstructions, changes in lifestyle were consistently more important in the amputee group. The mean annual hospital costs for the first four years were comparable. Slightly more than half of the amputees were retrained to a different profession and were drawing an extremely costly and lifelong invalidity pension compared to just below 20% of the reconstructed patients. They concluded that for potentially salvageable legs, reconstruction was advisable because the functional outcome was better, there was no permanent social disintegration due to the long treatment, and total costs (including pensions) for reconstruction were far lower than for amputation.

When amputation is necessary, Bondurant et al. (31) found that patients undergoing primary amputation had far fewer operations, shorter hospitalizations, and lower hospital costs than patients whose amputation was delayed a day or more after injury.

In summary, the treatment of the mangled extremity is fraught with difficulty, even for the most expert surgeon. The first necessity is recognizing the severity of the injury. At times, a threatened limb may initially present with a sensate foot with a pulse, yet crush, intimal injury and the possibility of muscle ischemia and delayed compartment syndrome can threaten the viability of the extremity. A high index of suspicion for threats to limb is crucial, because time lost can be catastrophic. The prompt institution of appropriate therapy produces the best results, but this can be difficult if subtle threats to the viability of the leg go unrecognized. For this reason, rapid transfer of patients with potentially limb-threatening injuries to centers with significant experience in their care is desirable.

Although Lange's criteria of division of the tibial nerve and prolonged warm ischemia time are probably the most accepted indications for amputation, even these are no longer absolute. Decision making is challenging, and currently takes place at a time when our largest, most comprehensive and most recent study has failed to validate the utility of any extremity injury-severity score (28). Certainly, if amputation is to be performed, it is better carried out promptly, but the choice is often unclear. It seems evident that the choice of reconstruction over amputation results in a greater number of procedures, a longer hospitalization, and greater costs in the short term, but it is unclear which carries the greater long-term costs, both financial and social. Current scoring systems provide a useful framework for decision making, but treatment must be individualized according to patient and family wishes. Additional patient-related variables outside the scoring systems, such as additional systemic injuries, smoking history, patient activity level, and vocational status should also be considered in decisions regarding potential limb salvage.

WOUND MANAGEMENT AND TIMING OF DEFINITIVE FIXATION

At the conclusion of the operative debridement, the surgeon proceeds with stabilization of the limb. It is desirable to perform the definitive fixation as soon as is safely possible, but judging the readiness of the limb for definitive repair is a complex process. The condition of patient (age, general health, single extremity or polytrauma, hemodynamic stability), the condition of extremity (swollen tissues, injured or abraded skin, zone of injury not clearly demarcated), the length and extent of the definitive procedure, the resources available, and the individual surgeon's philosophy and expertise all play a role in determining the timing of definitive osseous reconstruction. If the patient is sufficiently healthy, the procedure is not overlong, and the surgeon and institution are up to the task, the question becomes one of whether the patient and the limb are ready to undergo a surgical "second insult." At the present time, this is more a question of surgical philosophy than science, with the older literature advocating a delay prior to reconstruction, and the more recent literature showing that acute or early bony reconstruction and soft-tissue coverage often gives results which are superior to those obtained after a delay. More recently, there has been a partial swing back toward the older philosophy, with "early total care" being recommended only for patients without systemic injury, while "damage control orthopedics," is advocated for severely injured polytrauma victims to avoid the complications associated with prolonged operative times in patients with severe systemic injury (32). In the damage control system, early temporary stabilization is performed initially, with definitive stabilization deferred until the patient has recovered sufficiently from the systemic insult.

If the surgeon deems the limb unprepared for a definitive procedure, it must be stabilized temporarily. In the foot, ankle, tibia, and knee, this may often be accomplished with a simple splint. However, in cases of gross instability, rapid application of a temporary, bridging external fixator may be preferable. Fractures of the femoral shaft are not easily stabilized with splints and require traction or an external fixator if the patient's condition does not allow definitive fixation. If the patient's condition permits, intramedullary nailing of the femoral shaft is almost always the method of choice and offers advantages in terms of patient mobilization and ease of nursing care.

Central to the issue of timing definitive fixation is the condition of the soft tissues. To consider operations of any significant length, particularly for closed fractures that are to be fixed with open reduction and internal fixation, swelling must be sufficiently diminished so that the incisions can be created and closed without wound complications. It is abundantly clear that the longer the interval from trauma to surgery, the lower the incidence of wound problems, so the surgeon should not hurry to the operating room if there is any question that swelling may still be excessive. The reappearance of skin wrinkles at the surgical site is the sign that this has occurred. In the foot and ankle, in the leg, and at the knee, this usually takes at least a week, and may take as long as two to three. For intramedullary nailing of the tibia and femur, swelling is not a contraindication unless it is so severe that it raises the question of compartment syndrome. If a compartment syndrome is present or appears intraoperatively, it should be released promptly. If swelling is significant but compartment syndrome is absent, the procedure may be delayed to allow the swelling to abate, but the limb must be carefully monitored, and released if there is any sign compartment syndrome is developing.

Another consideration is the cleanliness of any open wound and the viability of the surrounding tissues. As previously mentioned, open fractures should be debrided in the operating room as soon as possible. If the wound is not significantly contaminated and the soft tissues healthy, or if the surgeon is confident about the debridement, definitive fixation may proceed and the wounds loosely closed primarily if soft-tissue swelling permits. Generally, this may be possible for Gustilo grades I and II and sometimes IIIA injuries. However, if there is gross contamination or severe soft-tissue injury, or one cannot be confident the debridement is complete, the wound can be temporarily covered and reassessed in the operating room, anywhere from 24 hours if the injury is severe to several days if the tissues appear healthy, and a definitive fixation will occur if swelling is sufficiently diminished.

One "tried and true" method of caring for highly contaminated wounds is to irrigate and debride them and then leave them open, begin dressing changes early on, and allow the wounds to either close by secondary intention, or to cover them with split thickness skin graft once a healthy bed of granulation tissue is present. This is certainly applicable to grades I to IIIA wounds, and may occasionally be an appropriate method for IIIC and some IIIB wounds prior to flap coverage. Recently, vacuum-assisted closure dressings, first reported in the German literature in 1996 (33), and popularized in the United States at Wake Forest University (34), provide closed suction and subatmospheric pressure over an open wound to speed the process of granulation tissue formation and facilitate secondary closure or prepare a bed for skin grafting.

With more severe open wounds, grade IIIB and many grade IIICs, flap coverage will be required. Beginning with Seligson (35), a number of authors have found a protocol utilizing antibiotic beads and plastic film to be useful in this situation. At the conclusion of the initial debridement, methylmethacrylate beads impregnated with enough antibiotic to elute high local concentrations are placed in the wound and covered with a porous plastic film. This provides a moist environment to prevent desiccation necrosis and concentrates the antibiotic locally to decrease the risk of infection. In their final series of 1085 consecutive compound limb fractures, Ostermann et al. (36) found an overall infection rate of 12% among 240 fractures which received only systemic antibiotic prophylaxis and a rate of 3.7% among 845 managed with the supplementary local use of aminoglycoside-polymethylmethacrylate beads. When the fractures were classified according to Gustilo, the statistically significant differences were found primarily in the more severe type IIIB and IIIC fractures. Although methylmethacrylate is the most common carrier for the antibiotic beads, hydroxyapatite, plaster of Paris, collagen sponges, and other carriers have also been used.

In grade IIIB and IIIC fractures, after the definitive fixation has been performed, the bone, soft-tissue structures, and hardware must be covered. Initial observations on these difficult fractures led to the conclusion that wounds should be left open, as primary closure was associated with a high rate of complications such as infection and nonunion. Gustilo et al. (1,2) observed this phenomenon in their early work as did Russell et al. (37), who found a high incidence of wound infection and delayed union after primary closure of open tibia fractures.

However, as the skill of plastic and microsurgeons has improved, there has been a trend toward earlier coverage of severe open fractures, with many, but not all, investigators reporting that early coverage of grade IIIB and IIIC wounds provides superior results in terms of infection rate, nonunion rates, time to union, length of hospitalization, and number of operative procedures.

Godina (38), in his classic work on early reconstruction of complex extremity trauma, reported on 532 patients who underwent microsurgical reconstruction following trauma to their extremities. Group 1 underwent free flap transfer within 72 hours of the injury, group 2 between 72 hours and three months of the injury, and group 3 at a mean of 3.4 years. Flap failure and infection rates were lower, bone healing times and length of hospitalization shorter, and number of operations fewer for the group receiving free flap coverage in less than 72 hours. (Flap failure rate was 0.75% in group 1, 12% in group 2, and 9.5% in group 3.) Postoperative infection occurred in 1.5% of group 1, 17.5% of group 2, and 6% of group 3. Bone-healing time was 6.8 months in group 1, 12.3 months in group 2, and 29 months in group 3. The average length of total hospital stay was 27 days for group 1, 130 days for group 2, and 256 days for group 3. The number of operations averaged 1.3 for group 1, 4.1 for group 2, and 7.8 for group 3.

In a similar experience, Cierny et al. (39), reviewing their experience with open tibial shaft fractures, found that with a treatment protocol based on early, aggressive wound management and fracture coverage utilizing muscle, myocutaneous, or free flap techniques, major and minor wound healing disturbances were found in 20.8% of the early (0–7 days) and 83.3% of the late (8–30 days) groups, with mean union times of 4.0 and 6.4 months, respectively.

In contrast, Yaremchuk et al. (40) reported on 22 lower extremity osteocutaneous defects managed with emergency debridement of devitalized soft tissue and bone, external fracture stabilization, and serial debridements to prepare the wound for closure with predominantly free-muscle transfers performed an average of 17 days (range 3–43 days) after injury. The early infection rate was 14%, two extremities were amputated, and there were no chronic infections.

More recently, Hertel et al. (41) reviewed 29 consecutive open fractures of the tibia, including 24 grade IIIB and, five grade IIIC fractures, treated using a protocol of immediate debridement, early definitive skeletal stabilization, and early soft-tissue reconstruction. Fifteen were reconstructed after a mean delay of four days, whereas 14 were reconstructed immediately as an emergency procedure. Groups were comparable for sex, age, type of trauma, associated general injuries, type of fracture, associated arterial lesion, associated tendon rupture, type of soft-tissue reconstruction, and duration of follow-up. At a mean follow-up of 47 months, in the delayed reconstruction group, the time to unprotected weight bearing, time to definitive union, number of reoperations, and infection rate were significantly higher.

Gopal et al. (42) reviewed 84 consecutive patients with severe (Gustilo IIIB or IIIC) open fracture of the tibia treated by an immediate radical debridement of the wound and skeletal stabilization and early soft-tissue cover with a vascularized muscle flap. Stabilization of the fracture was achieved with 19 external and 65 internal fixation devices (nails or plates). Three patients required bone-transport procedures. Fifty-one fractures (66%) progressed to primary bony union and 26 (34%) required a bone-stimulating procedure. There was a rate of serious pin-track infection in 37% in the external fixator group. Treatment of these injuries by this aggressive combined approach provided good results. Immediate internal fixation and healthy soft-tissue cover with a muscle flap was safe. Delay in cover (>72 hours) was associated with most of the problems. External fixation was associated with practical difficulties for the plastic surgeons, chronic pin-track infections, and the only cases of malunion.

In a similar but smaller series, Sinclair et al. (43) reviewed 17 consecutive patients with grade IIIB open tibial fractures with treatment of both the fracture and the soft tissues performed with free tissue transfer within 72 hours of injury. There were no deep infections, flap survival of 100%, and mean time to fracture healing of 10 months.

In summary, it appears to be safe to close grade I and II and some IIIA wounds primarily after an adequate debridement, provided no gross contamination is present. If the wounds are contaminated, debridement followed by either open wound or bead pouch management with additional debridement prior to closure should be adequate. When trauma leaves significant soft tissue and bone deficiencies, regional or free flap reconstruction is necessary. The majority of the recent literature suggests that achieving this coverage within a few days time will result in better outcomes and fewer complications; however, when the patient's condition or other circumstances prevent this, excellent results are still possible if surgeons follow the principle of achieving adequate debridement prior to performing flap coverage. Once sufficient soft-tissue coverage is present, repair of fractures and reconstruction of bone deficiencies may be performed.

MANAGEMENT OF BONE LOSS

A further problem often encountered in the setting of the severely traumatized limb is the loss of bone stock. Gross contamination, devascularization, and actual loss of bone at the site of trauma in the field all present additional challenges to the orthopedic surgeon. When the bone loss includes the articular surface, difficulties achieving joint stability and the threat of posttraumatic arthritis challenge the orthopedist. Situations where there is significant diaphyseal loss present challenges to union, and, in cases of severe loss, force the surgeon to choose between shortening the limb or undertaking a lengthy course of limb lengthening, extensive cancellous grafting, or intercalary grafting to restore a limb of appropriate length.

Articular Surface

Deficiencies of the articular surface are extremely difficult to reconstruct. When a fracture involves the joint surface, osteoarticular fragments that have lost all blood supply may be present. When fractures are either closed or open, but not grossly contaminated, these fragments may be incorporated into the repair of the joint surface. Only in cases of the severest contamination or unreconstructable comminution should portions of the articular surface be discarded. At other times, there may be actual loss of portions of the articular surface at the site of injury. In these situations, where the joint surface either cannot be repaired, or is not present, the surgeon is faced with a difficult choice between repairing the portion of the joint that remains, and accepting that result, or performing an immediate joint fusion. In rare circumstances, once soft tissues have been reconstructed and there is no evidence of infection, partial or entire joint surfaces may be reconstructed or salvaged with large osteoarticular allograft transplants (44).

Diaphyseal

Loss of diaphyseal bone also presents a reconstructive challenge. Unlike the cancellous bone on osteoarticular fragments, devascularized segments of the diaphysis have poor potential for healing, present a potential focus for infection, and are not vital to the ultimate reconstruction of the limb. In cases of moderate diaphyseal loss, sufficient bone may remain for union to occur. It may be possible to fix the bone at its original length and bone graft the defect early with cancellous bone or to treat with a reamed exchange nailing in the femur or tibia. In other instances, in may be possible to shorten the bone slightly in order to obtain bone-to-bone contact. However, in cases where the bone loss is severe, the treating surgeon must either accept significant shortening of the limb, or provide a means for reconstituting its length. Although there are case reports of replantation of large devascularized diaphyseal segments, this should be attempted only by very experienced surgeons and with the greatest caution because of the extremely high risk of infection and nonunion.

Numerous techniques have been employed to regain length in cases of diaphyseal bone loss. Two basic treatment strategies exist. The first consists of acute shortening followed by a period of limb lengthening; the second involves fixing the extremity at the appropriate length and using either bone transport, bone grafting, or free vascularized bone transfers to fill in the defect. Typically, the soft tissues are allowed to heal prior to filling in the bone defect, but more recently, some have begun performing immediate bone grafting and soft-tissue coverage. In all cases, it is crucial that the initial fracture care include meticulous debridement of all devitalized soft tissue and diaphyseal bone, and that a competent soft-tissue envelope be established to accommodate the reconstruction.

The technique of acute shortening followed by a period of limb lengthening is usually performed according to the principles of Ilizarov (45). After a thorough debridement, including the removal of devitalized bone, the fracture ends are brought together. An external fixator is then applied, a corticotomy made away from the zone of injury, and lengthening carried out through the corticotomy. Compression at the fracture brings about union, and simultaneous distraction restores limb length. Others (46) have allowed fracture healing to take place after the primary shortening, and begun distraction 6 to 12 months after injury. These methods of acute shortening may help decrease the need for free soft-tissue transfers to obtain bone coverage. As an alternative, some authors (47) have brought the bone ends that remain viable together and distracted through the fracture once callus formation has begun.

Numerous authors have described methods of fixing the extremity at its appropriate length and reconstituting the bone stock. As always, a complete debridement is necessary to decrease risk of infection or systemic injury and to provide a viable soft-tissue envelope. If necessary, local or free flap coverage occurs once complete debridement has been achieved. One of the classic ways to restore bone is to transport a segment of bone from a proximal corticotomy down into the bone defect. Compression at the site where the transported segment "docks" into the distal bone heals the docking site. In the gap where the transported segment has moved away from the proximal bone, a mass of regenerate bone forms and consolidates. Although a thin wire fixator is typically used, half pin or unilateral fixators and distraction over an intramedullary nail are also used.

Other techniques include vascularized transfer of either the ipsilateral or the contralateral fibula, or the iliac crest (48). Also reported is a technique of tibialization of the fibula by transporting it utilizing an adaptation of the Ilizarov technique (49). Other authors, such as Christian et al. (50), have described excellent results with massive allografting of traumatic defects averaging 10 cm in length.

More recently, a number of authors have described the acute reconstruction of soft tissue and bony defects following severe trauma. Hertel et al. (30), Tropet et al. (51), and Musharrafieh et al. (52) have all reported on the emergent bony and soft-tissue reconstruction of contaminated fractures with high rates of bone union, low rates of complications, and a small number of hospitalizations and operative procedures required relative to delayed reconstructions.

The following case demonstrates creative use of several of the above principles to solve a difficult clinical problem (courtesy James J. Hutson, MD). A postman and part-time plumber fell into a septic tank and sustained an open distal tibial fracture (Fig. 5). He was treated with emergent irrigation, debridement, and placement of a temporary ankle-spanning external fixator (Fig. 6), that was converted to an Ilizarov-type frame once the soft tissues appeared healthy (Fig. 7). Despite this appropriate care, he developed a severe deep infection. He was treated utilizing surgical principles similar to those used for grossly contaminated open fractures. All devitalized tissues, including a large portion of the distal tibial articular surface tissues were debrided, leaving a large void (Fig. 8), which was then packed with methylmethacrylate antibiotic beads (Figs. 9 and 10). When the infection was controlled, the end of the remaining distal tibial shaft was contoured to the shape of the articular surface and the limb acutely shortened to make a new ankle joint (Fig. 11). Several years later, the ankle is healed with no infection (Fig. 12). The patient wears a shoe lift (Fig. 13), has partial ankle motion with little pain, and continues to work full time as a postman.

METHODS OF FRACTURE FIXATION

A detailed description of the techniques of fracture fixation is beyond the scope of this chapter. Beginning with the femoral shaft and moving down to the foot, we present a summary of the timing of fixation, operative approach, and preferred methods of fixation. In long-bone fractures, the surgeon's aim is to restore limb

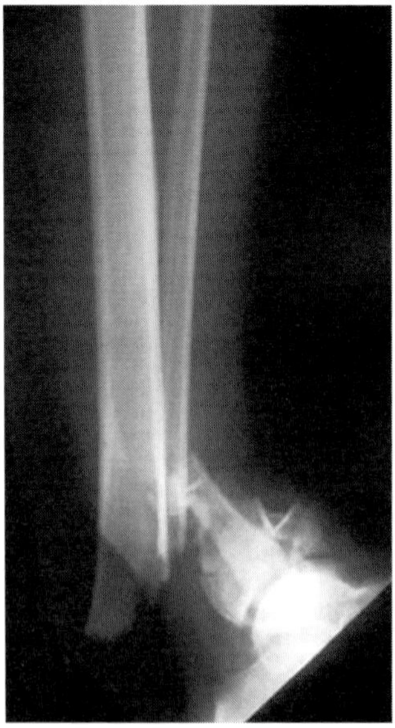

Figure 5 Open distal tibia fracture due to a fall into a septic tank.

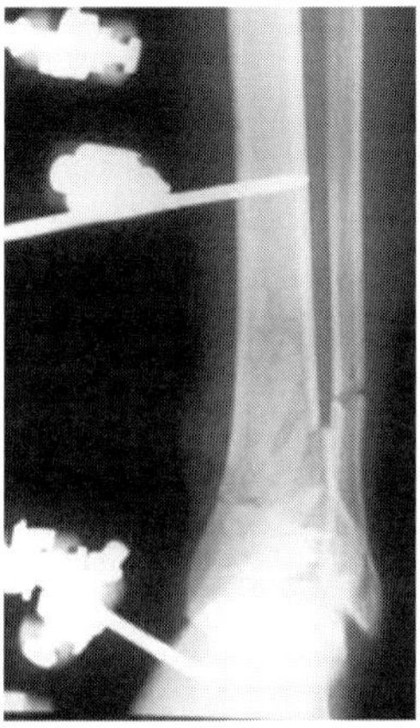

Figure 6 Post-debridement temporary external fixation of the injury shown above.

axis, length, and rotation. For articular fractures, the goal is to restore congruent joint surfaces, preferably with enough stability to permit early range of motion. For a more thorough discussion of the principles of fracture fixation, the reader is referred to one of the two definitive English language texts, *Skeletal Trauma* (53) or *Rockwood, Green and Wilkins' Fractures* (54).

Femoral Shaft Fractures

The shaft of the femur is stout, cylindrical, and capable of withstanding significant loads. The amount of force necessary for failure in nonpathologic adult bone

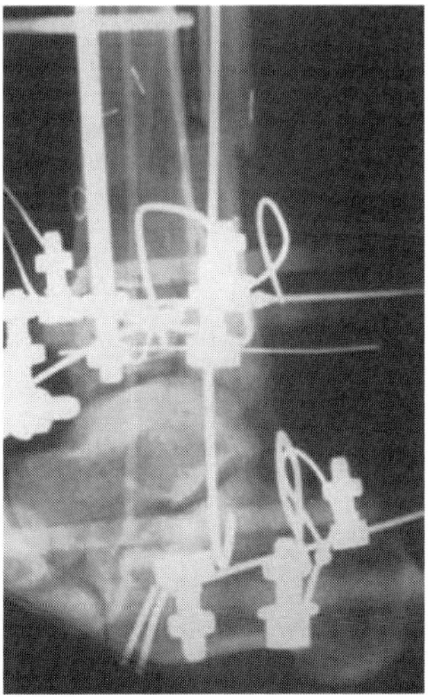

Figure 7 Initial definitive fixation of injury shown in Figure 5.

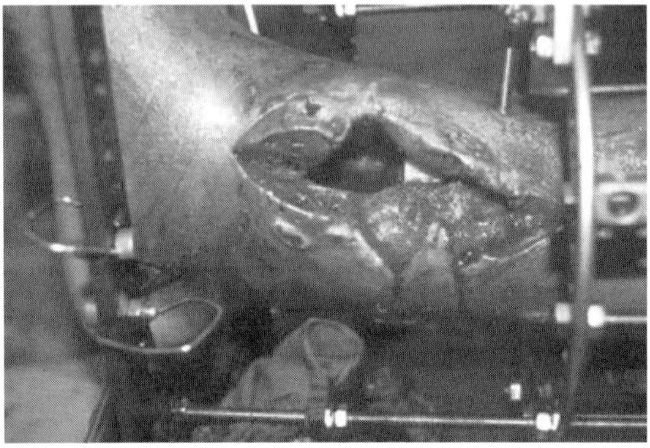

Figure 8 The patient developed infection. His distal tibia was necrotic and was debrided leaving a large void.

is generally attained only with events such as motor vehicle accidents and falls from great heights (55,56). Because of the massive energy required, fractures of the shaft of the femur have significant associated morbidities—from both the femoral injury itself and from other systemic injuries from the traumatic event. It is critical that the treating facility be capable of managing both the injury and the untoward events occasionally encountered with femur fractures, such as fat embolism and pulmonary embolism (57). In addition, the facility should also be equipped to treat the other life-threatening injuries frequently sustained from such violent events. Initial evaluation should be in accordance with advanced trauma life-support guidelines. Recognition of the potential for significant hemorrhage is essential, and adequate fluid resuscitation should follow.

Once hemodynamic stability has been established, careful examination of the afflicted extremity is conducted. Assessment of the limb's neurovascular status, and a search for other injuries, particularly in the hip and knee, are of paramount importance. When the survey of the limb is completed, in-line skeletal

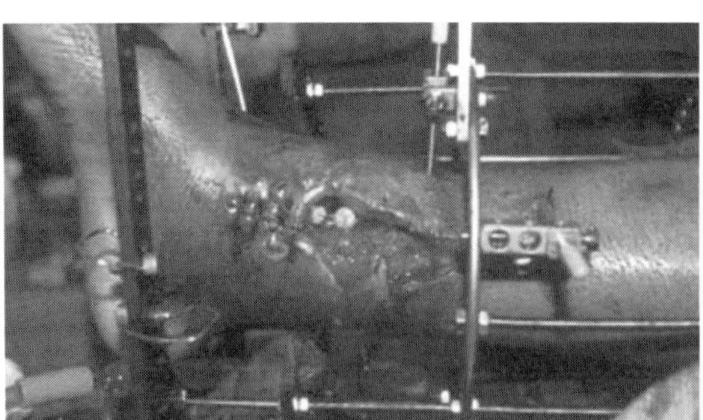

Figure 9 The void was filled with antibiotic-ladon methylmethacrylate beads until soft tissue coverage was obtained.

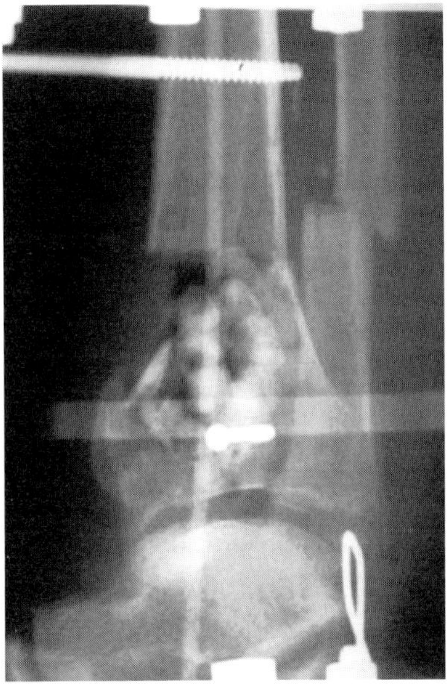

Figure 10 Antibiotic beads in place filling a large void.

traction with approximately 25 pounds is applied via a pin placed through either the proximal tibia or the distal femur. Abrasions and lacerations are inspected for possible communication with an underlying fracture. Owing to the robust circumferential envelope of muscle, the majority of these fractures are closed. When the fractures do communicate with an overlying wound, they are generally classified

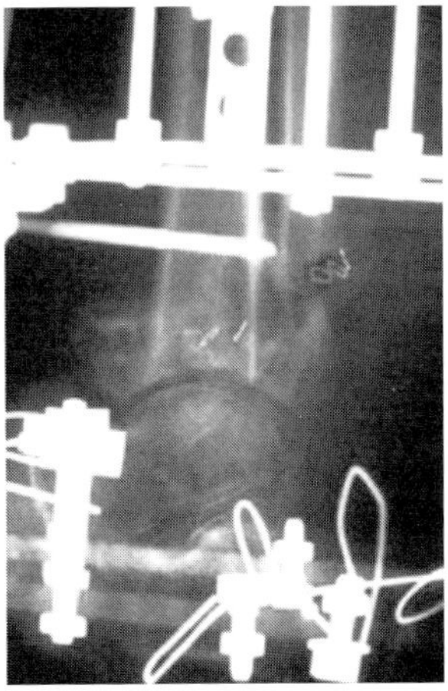

Figure 11 The remaining distal tibia was contoured to the shape of the distal tibia and the leg shortened to make a "new" ankle joint.

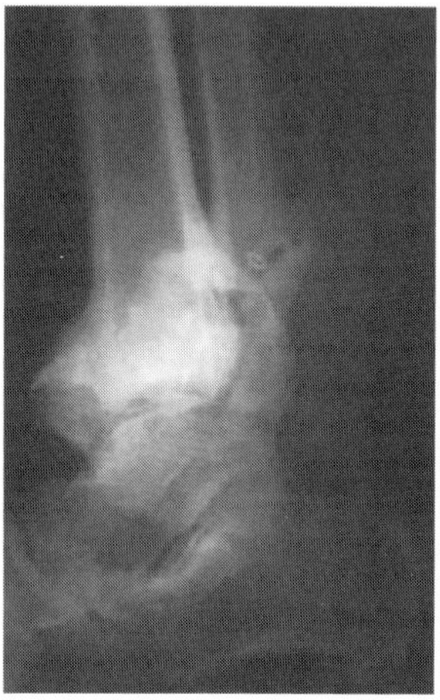

Figure 12 Years later, the joint is healed without infection.

according to Gustilo et al. (2). Open fractures are treated with emergent irrigation and debridement, and either definitive internal or temporary external fixation as the patient's condition allows.

Historically, these patients were definitively treated with casting or traction devices. The test of time proved these modalities suboptimal due to a high incidence of complications (58), and modern techniques of internal fixation are now the standard of care. For acute, closed femoral shaft fractures, the definitive treatment of choice is almost always internal fixation with an intramedullary nail. The

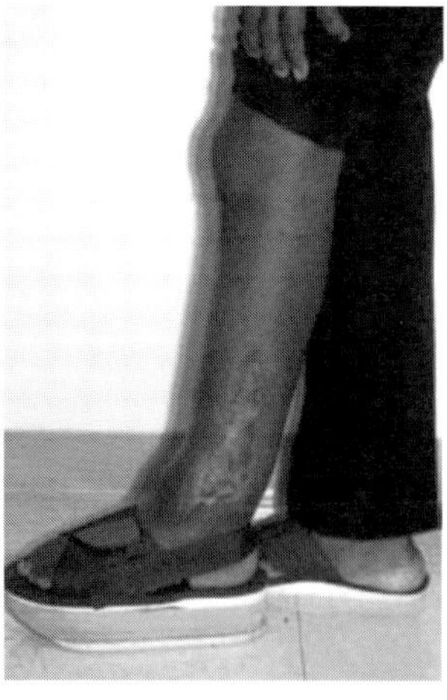

Figure 13 Patient has little pain, walks with a shoe lift, and works as a postman.

same is true of most open fractures that have been meticulously debrided and given prophylactic antibiotics (59,60). Plate and screw fixation has diminished in popularity as nailing techniques have improved, but still remains a viable option in some circumstances. Because the investing layer of muscle is circumferential along the entire shaft, soft-tissue coverage is rarely a problem. Only in cases of massive contamination or devastating muscle loss do the soft tissues preclude nailing.

Originally popularized by Kuntscher (61), intramedullary fixation may now be inserted in an antegrade fashion through the greater trochanter or piriformis fossa, or in a retrograde fashion through the knee. With the advent of percutaneous techniques and fluoroscopic guidance, this can typically be accomplished with 1-inch incisions and minimal disturbance of the surrounding soft tissues. It is now customary to ream the medullary canal to allow a slightly larger rod to better "fit" the canal of the femur, and to statically lock the nail with screws inserted transversely through the nail both above and below the fracture site. This prevents additional muscle damage by stabilizing the limb, promotes early mobilization, and facilitates patient transport, nursing care, and access to the soft tissues. In large series, both early and recent (62,63) complication rates are low, and union rates are well above 90%.

Although intramedullary is almost always preferred, there are times when other forms of fixation are more appropriate. For some type IIIB and type IIIC fractures, external fixation may be the best option (64,65). Intramedullary nailing in these instances has a higher rate of infection, and the time and physical nature of inserting the intramedullary rod also makes it less desirable when the muscle envelope is severely damaged, or when an immediate vascular repair is necessary for limb salvage. In experienced hands, external fixation requires less than 30 minutes and affords enough stability for transfers and ambulation with protected weight-bearing, and simplifies wound care. External fixation can also be used for femoral shaft fractures in critically ill patients not physiologically suited to undergo a definitive procedure. Half pins inserted into the femur are inserted from either anterior or lateral both above and below the fracture and connected with clamps, and bars align and stabilize the bone fragments. The fixator stabilizes the fracture without causing the potential pulmonary insult that can occur during nail insertion, and may be left as definitive fixation, or used as a temporary bridge to a later internal fixation. If a long period of time passes before conversion from external fixation to an intramedullary nail, the medullary canal should be considered contaminated, and the risk of infection may be significantly increased (66). In these cases, the external fixator is often best left in place until healing has occurred.

Supracondylar Femur Fractures

Fractures of the metaphysis and articular surface of the distal femur present a challenge to the orthopedic surgeon. These fractures have a bimodal distribution, occurring after high-energy trauma in young adults and after lower-energy falls in geriatric patients with osteoporotic bone. In the young, accompanying soft-tissue injuries can be severe. In the elderly, the soft tissues are less resilient, but the degree of injury is often less severe. Fortunately, injuries of the distal femur usually benefit from the robust soft-tissue envelope of the thigh, making the need for flap coverage rare. However, high-energy injuries about the knee do carry with them the additional risk of accompanying vascular injury.

Emergency department management begins with a systematic and thorough evaluation of the patient. Cardiac and cerebrovascular events should be considered as potential etiology of falls in the elderly, and may in fact present a greater threat than the skeletal injury. When a high-energy mechanism is present, local neurovascular injury and other associated life-threatening injuries from the trauma should be sought out and dealt with appropriately. When the survey of the extremity is complete, the limb should be placed in a knee immobilizer if there is little skeletal deformity or shortening, or placed in either proximal or distal tibial traction if significant shortening exists.

In the setting of an open fracture or a vascular injury, emergent surgical intervention is required. Open fractures should be meticulously debrided in the operating room and then either temporary or definitive fixation carried out. In the case of vascular injury, an external fixator may be rapidly applied in order to stabilize the limb, so that the vascular repair may be performed on a stable leg. When the repair is complete, the knee may be straightened while the repair is visualized directly to verify that it remains patent.

A distinguishing feature of external fixators applied in this situation is the need to span the knee. Half pins are placed in the femoral and tibial diaphyses to form a stable base on either side of the knee, and the fracture is then pulled to length on rods connecting the two sides of the joint. These "bridge" frames serve as portable traction devices, allow access to the limb for wound care, facilitate patient mobilization, and maintain gross limb alignment while the soft tissues recover to a state sufficient to permit a safe definitive skeletal repair.

Radiographic survey generally demonstrates a characteristic apex posterior deformity of the fracture at the supracondylar level, due to the unopposed pull of the gastrocnemius muscles on the posterior aspect of the femoral condyles, and the deforming forces of the quadriceps and hamstrings across the fracture and the knee joint itself. Skeletal traction followed by cast bracing was historically used as definitive treatment (67,68) but is now employed very infrequently. Beginning in the 1970s, numerous publications of improved techniques of reduction and fixation appeared, with reports of superior results (69–71). The capacity to achieve near anatomic reduction of the articular surface, reproduce and maintain the mechanical and anatomic axes, and begin early motion has proven monumental in minimizing the posttraumatic arthritis and arthrofibrosis seen in patients treated with earlier techniques.

Definitive fixation can be carried out within the first few hours after injury if the patient is physiologically suited, the limb is not grossly contaminated, and the appropriate operating facilities are available. Otherwise, open fractures should be debrided and the limb placed in either skeletal traction or a bridge frame until swelling has diminished to a point where the definitive surgery can be carried out safely. If the articular surface and metaphysis are intact, or are merely split and can be fixed anatomically with one or two screws, the fracture may often be fixed with a retrograde intramedullary nail, which minimizes soft-tissue dissection (72,73).

If significant articular comminution is present, the definitive repair begins with open reduction and internal fixation of the articular surface. Once this has been accomplished, the articular surface is fixed to the shaft of the femur with the appropriate axis, length, and rotation. This is generally accomplished with a fixed angle plate and screw construct. Until recently, blade plates and the dynamic condylar screw were most popular. However, recent designs which provide screws that lock to the plates at fixed angles, with devices that allow a near percutaneous insertion (74) are proving both popular and efficacious (75,76). Union rates approach 95% to 98%, and rates of malunion and infection are low. Knee motion, though improved with these modalities, remains a significant obstacle to these patients, particularly in the elderly.

In situations where the soft tissues are too damaged to provide coverage for plate and screw fixation, or in situations where the amount of articular or periarticular comminution make it impossible to obtain fixation stable enough to allow early motion, definitive or supplemental treatment with external fixation presents a viable alternative (77,78). When the articular surfaces can be fixed, but not so well that they are stable, it is very reasonable to protect the fixation by bridging the knee for several weeks, then remove the fixator under anesthesia and manipulate the knee to improve motion. When plate and screw fixation is not possible, the bridge frame can be left on until the fracture is healed, but this can lead to stiffness that may require an operative release.

Proximal Tibia Fractures

As with supracondylar fractures of the femur, proximal tibia fractures occur in a bimodal distribution, generally as a consequence of high-energy trauma in the young and low-energy falls in the elderly. Among the elderly, this fracture receives much attention because it is a common injury, accounting for 8% of all fractures in this age group, and potentially causing significant functional impairment (79). Among younger patients, this injury can occur as the result of a more forceful axial load, or as a result of devastatingly high-energy trauma, such as that imparted by the bumper of a car. As the tibia is a largely subcutaneous bone, the fracture is more likely to be open than those of the distal femur, and more likely to have internal degloving and periosteal stripping—all factors that weigh heavily when determining the timing and method of fixation.

An axial load with a concomitant valgus or varus stress about the knee typically results in failure of the proximal portion of the tibia. The outcome is usually a combination of depression and splitting of the articular surface. The Schatzker et al. (80) classification, first described in 1979, is most commonly used today. Types I–III involve either splitting and/or depression of the lateral plateau.

Type IV involves the medial plateau and is often a knee dislocation equivalent, carrying a significant risk of associated vascular and ligamentous injury. Types V and VI, which usually follow higher-energy injury, consist of injury to both medial and lateral plateaus, without (type V) or with (type VI) dissociation of the entire metaphyseal portion from the shaft.

Evaluation of the patient should be meticulous. Because these fractures occur where the common peroneal nerve wraps around the fibular neck, and where the popliteal artery trifurcates into the anterior and posterior tibial and peroneal arteries, associated nerve and vascular injuries are common. These injuries, along with the possibility of accompanying compartment syndrome, should be sought in all proximal tibial fractures. Ligamentous and meniscal injury are also common, and may be found in as many as 30% and 50% of the cases, respectively (81). Plain radiographs of the knee and the femoral and tibial shaft should be obtained. Computerized tomography (CT) scans with multiplanar reconstructions are useful for determining the specific architecture of the fracture and the best surgical approach, and should be obtained for all but the most simple fractures. The use of magnetic resonance imaging is not routine, although some have recommended its use for evaluation of the menisci and ligaments.

In cases of vascular injury, conventional angiography or the newer CT or magnetic resonance angiography are desirable studies. However, the surgeon should remember that a vascular injury at the knee is a limb-threatening emergency and that urgent surgical correction is of paramount importance. Unless the formal study is immediately available, or the limb is traumatized at multiple levels, an emergent trip to the operating room for on-table angiography and surgical exploration may be more prudent.

For closed, nondisplaced or minimally displaced fractures, closed treatment is still advocated. While there is no clear consensus on a specific, acceptable amount of displacement of the articular surface, "minimal" is generally taken to mean 2 or 3 mm. Immobilization of the knee with either a long leg cast or a hinged knee immobilizer is prescribed for approximately four to six weeks. When the fracture is though to be "sticky," gentle range of motion is begun. After 8 to 12 weeks of nonweight bearing, the patient begins gradual, progressive, protected weight bearing until a full unassisted gait is attained. Surveillance radiographs should be obtained during the rehabilitation phase to rule out loss of reduction. The most commonly cited complications are arthrofibrosis secondary to prolonged immobilization and knee pain from posttraumatic arthritis.

When there is significant incongruity of the joint surface or angulation of the limb, or when the fracture is open, surgical treatment is indicated. The timing of surgery is dictated by the condition of the surrounding soft tissues. For closed injuries that require open reduction and internal fixation, the decision is usually made based upon the amount of swelling present. Fractures at the proximal portion of the tibia have the propensity to swell to such an extent that they may cause blistering of the skin. Incisions through these compromised locations carry with them an elevated risk of problems with wound closure and wound healing, creating an increased risk of infection. Hardware left exposed holds an unacceptably high rate of deep infection and should be avoided.

If a skin defect communicates with an underlying fracture, the standard of care is formal debridement within six to eight hours from injury. Lacerations around the knee may represent an open joint and should be evaluated by injection of a large bolus (60 cm^3) of sterile saline into the knee joint through intact tissues. Extravasation of fluid from the wound indicates an open joint that should be debrided and lavaged in the operating room.

The decision as to whether or not to temporarily or definitively fix the fracture at the time of initial debridement is based on the time since injury, amount of contamination, soft-tissue loss, and swelling. Gustilo–Anderson types I–IIIA are often amenable to conventional open reduction and internal fixation with plate and screws at the conclusion of a meticulous debridement, if the patient has made it to the operating room before the onset of significant swelling. If contamination, soft-tissue loss, or swelling preclude definitive fixation, the wound should be irrigated and debrided, and the joint bridged with a simple half pin fixator spanning the knee. This serves to maintain length and aid in reduction by way of ligamentotaxis, and allows time and protection for soft-tissue recovery or demarcation. If it is possible without additional dissection distal into the leg, the articular surface may be fixed at this time. Formal plating should be deferred until swelling is largely resolved. At that time, an arthrotomy combined with longitudinal incisions allows visualization, reduction, and internal fixation of both the articular surfaces and the articular segment to the tibial shaft.

With less invasive techniques, definitive fixation may be possible even in the face of significant swelling. The articular surface is reduced with either mini-incisions or arthroscopic or fluoroscopic assistance. The articular surface is then aligned to the shaft and fixed with either an external fixator, or with newer locked plates designed to be inserted percutaneously. Either a hybrid fixator (which attaches a fine-wire ring to the plateau and connects it to half pins in the shaft) or an Ilizarov-type fixator allows the surgeon to maintain limb axis, alignment, and rotation without the dissection necessary to place a plate and screws. This is a particularly attractive option when the plateau fracture is associated with comminution of the shaft, and has the additional benefit of allowing earlier weight bearing than plate and screw constructs. Newer-generation intramedullary nails, with screws that interlock proximally at multiple heights and angles, have extended the indications for use of intramedullary devices for plateau fractures associated with fractures of the proximal shaft, but are still only suitable for relatively simple articular patterns.

Tibial Shaft Fractures

Tibial shaft fractures are among the most common long-bone injuries (82). Like femoral diaphyseal fractures, the goal when managing these injuries is to reestablish and maintain the correct axial alignment, length, and rotation of the limb, while facilitating the patient's rehabilitation. Although no absolute guidelines exist, angulation or rotation of 5° to 10° and shortening of 1–2 cm are generally considered the upper limits of acceptable deviation from normal alignment. Although it is unproven, some suspect that changing limb alignment beyond this degree could alter joint contact forces in both the knee and the ankle and lead to premature arthrosis. However, no study has yet demonstrated untoward clinical effects as a result of minor degrees of malalignment.

Tibial shaft fractures of minor severity (low energy, minimal comminution, closed, or minimally open, with shortening of less than 1.5 cm and displacement of less than 50% of the shaft width) are generally considered suitable for cast treatment. Closed reduction and casting can correct angulation and rotation, but usually cannot correct shortening or displacement. Those fractures which cannot be well maintained in a cast, as well as most tibial shaft fractures of greater severity, should be treated surgically—generally with a reamed, locked intramedullary nail (4).

Patients are initially placed into a long leg cast with the knee in almost full extension and permitted weight bearing to tolerance. Once the patient is able to ambulate comfortably, the cast is exchanged for a removable fracture brace and assistive devices weaned. In series of appropriately selected patients, this technique demonstrates union rates from 95% to 100%, with an average of less than eight degrees of angulation, and little shortening beyond that demonstrated on the initial injury film (83,84). Proponents of functional fracture bracing note both a high union rate and freedom from surgical complications in support of this technique. However, this method of treatment is labor intensive, requiring frequent X rays, occasional remanipulations and cast changes, and a compliant patient. In contrast, operative intervention allows the surgeon to achieve and maintain near anatomic reduction, while allowing an earlier and easier rehabilitation.

Inherently unstable fractures (85,86) (greater than 50% comminution of the cortical circumference, or 50% displacement), open fractures, and fractures in polytrauma patients are generally treated with some type of internal fixation. In the vast majority of cases, this takes the form of an intramedullary nail. However, in some cases, plate and screw fixation, percutaneous plating, or external fixation with either half pin or fine-wire frames may be appropriate.

Emergency department evaluation begins with the usual primary and secondary surveys of the severely injured patient. The value of a thorough neurovascular exam cannot be overemphasized. A high-energy mechanism of injury should alert the physician to look beyond the obvious fracture for soft-tissue injury as well, as this has significant therapeutic and prognostic implications. In addition to the obvious open fracture, soft-tissue injuries may include deep contaminated skin abrasions, significant muscle crush, internal degloving, neurovascular injury, and impending or established compartment syndrome. Tscherne's classification for closed fractures (5), described in detail above, is helpful in determining both the nature and the timing of treatment.

Closed unstable fractures should be temporarily stabilized with well-padded plaster splints in order to prevent additional insult and maximize patient comfort. In those fractures classified as Tscherne C0 (negligible) or C1 (mild to moderate), soft-tissue injury may be fixed definitively within the first 24 hours. Modern statically locked intramedullary rods have yielded union rates as high as 100% and infection rates of 0.9% to 6% in these circumstances (4,87) CII (significant) and CIII (severe) soft-tissue injuries should have their definitive surgery delayed until soft tissues have demarcated and edema diminished so that complications such as wound dehiscence and infection can be minimized (88). This may require from a few days to over a week before a definitive procedure can be undertaken safely. Temporary stabilization with an external fixator during this interim aids the process of soft-tissue recovery, but requires an additional operation, and carries a risk of pin site infection that can increase the risk of deep infection following the definitive repair.

Open fractures should be taken to the operating room within six to eight hours from injury for exploration, irrigation, and meticulous debridement. In most cases, Gustilo type I, II, IIIA open fractures may be fixed with an intramedullary nail at that time. The majority of fracture surgeons use either a tight-fitting nail inserted without reaming or ream lightly in order to improve nail fit. In cases of type IIIB fractures, with severe soft-tissue injury that will generally require flap coverage, treatment is controversial. Immediate nailing is possible, but requires a radical debridement with either immediate or early coverage. If flap coverage cannot be obtained promptly, the risk of infection and treatment failure rises and other treatments should be considered. In type IIIC fractures, the first step is deciding whether or not to attempt limb salvage. If the limb is to be saved, the patient must move promptly to the operating room for temporary stabilization and revascularization.

In these most severe injuries, external fixation is the short-term treatment of choice in the majority of cases. Generally, this takes the form of an anterior half-pin frame, which will bridge to the foot if the shaft fracture extends distally. The frame is generally left in place until revascularization and/or flap coverage is safely established. At that time, the patient may be converted to definitive nail or plate fixation. In some circumstances, the frame may be left in place as the definitive treatment. However, this form of treatment is generally associated with slower fracture healing and late loss of alignment if the frame is converted to cast treatment before the fracture is completely healed (84).

In centers with expertise in their use, ring fixators of the type described by Ilizarov provide an excellent alternative treatment to these most difficult fractures. In expert hands, thin wire fixators can be applied either immediately or in a delayed fashion, before, at, or after the time of flap coverage. They have a low rate of infection, are the least disturbing to the remaining soft-tissue attachments of the bone, and produce high union rates. Because they require no deep or permanent hardware, they can be used to treat even IIIB fractures successfully without resorting to the usual flap coverage (89). The frames can be used to obtain and maintain reduction, and often permit immediate weight-bearing during the patient's recovery. In circumstances where there is significant bone loss, the

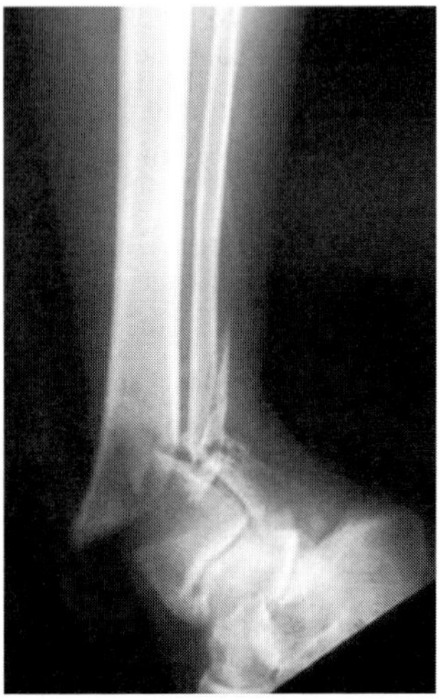

Figure 14 A high-energy distal tibia fracture.

frame can be used to make up these defects by transporting bone across the area of loss until union has been obtained.

The following demonstrates the use of an Ilizarov fixator to treat a IIIB open distal tibial fracture without flap coverage (again courtesy of James J. Hutson, MD). A middle-aged male in a motor vehicle accident sustained this open distal tibial fracture (Fig. 14). Although the wound is not large, skin loss over the anteromedial distal tibia presents an extremely difficult problem (Fig. 15). The plate that would typically be placed through this zone of injury to fix the fracture would almost inevitably become infected if it were not urgently covered by a local or free flap. Managing the fracture with an Ilizarov frame and the wound with dressing changes

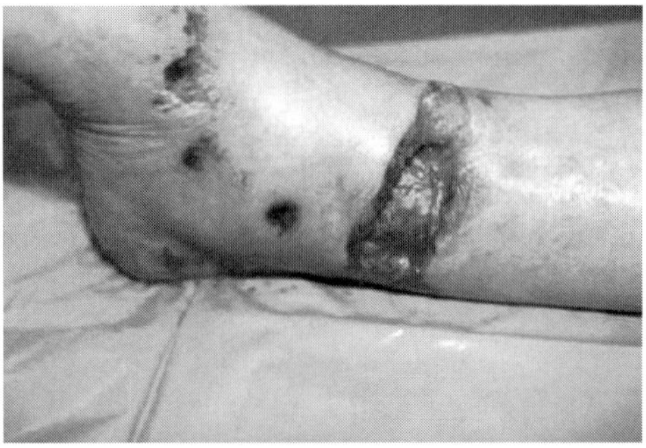

Figure 15 The clinical photo shows the skin loss. Although the wound is small, the anteromedial tibia typically presents severe coverage problems.

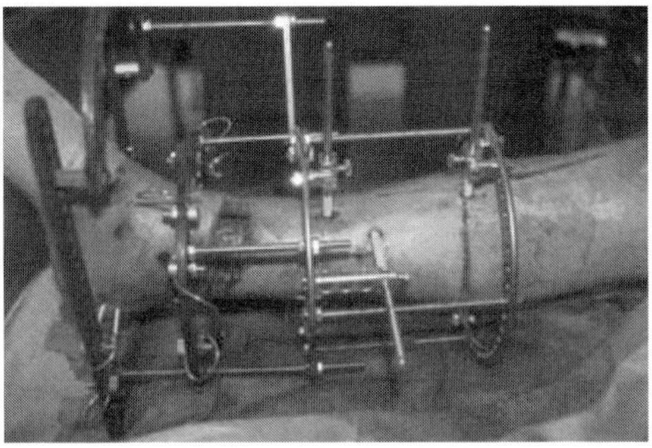

Figure 16 The Ilizarov frame in place.

allows both fracture healing and wound healing by secondary intention with no flap coverage and no deep infection (Figs. 16–19).

Distal Tibia Fractures

Fractures of the distal tibia (the tibial pilon) and its articular surface (the plafond), while rare, are notoriously difficult injuries whose treatment is fraught with complications. Although they comprise less than 10% of all tibia fractures, they are frequently high-energy, open injuries with contamination, crush of the soft-tissue envelope, and degloving of the underlying bone. Articular comminution, metaphyseal impaction, and damage to the cartilage surfaces, coupled with severe soft-tissue injury, make fractures of the tibial pilon injuries which can easily result in amputation. Salvage of severe distal tibia fractures is almost an art in and of itself, and should only be undertaken by the most skilled of surgeons.

The mechanism of injury is usually a combination of axial load and rotation of the talus on the articular surface of the distal tibia. When torsional forces, such as those that occur in sports such as skiing, cause the injury, the fractures

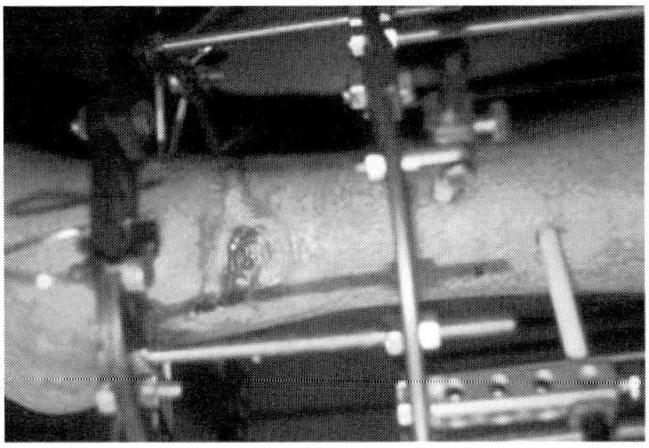

Figure 17 The wound granulating with dressing changes.

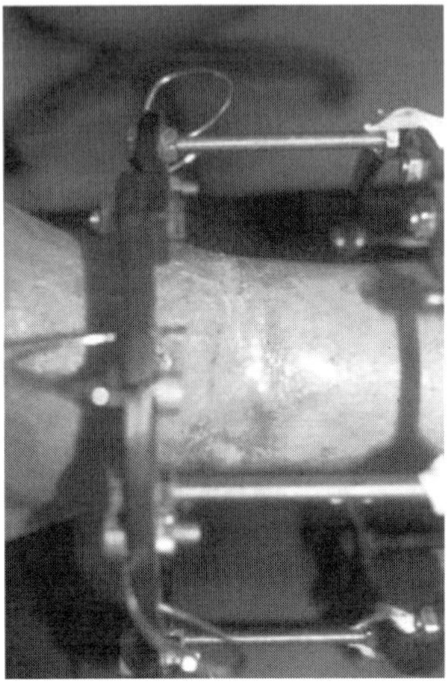

Figure 18 The wound—healed.

tend to be lower energy, with less articular comminution and less soft-tissue damage. Not surprisingly, these fractures have better outcomes and fewer complications. When axial forces predominate, the loads involved can be tremendous. High-energy trauma, such as a fall from a height or a motorcycle accident or car

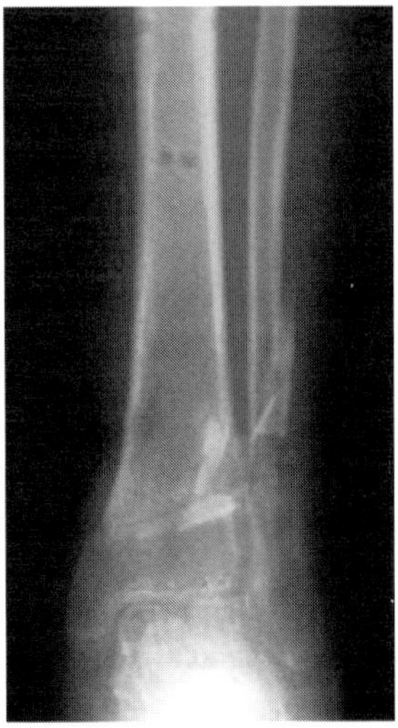

Figure 19 The fracture—healed.

accident with a sudden stop, can cause such articular, metaphyseal, and soft-tissue injury that saving the limb may difficult, if not impossible.

Initial evaluation of the patient in the emergency department should include careful scrutiny of the entire patient as well as the affected limb. Because these fractures are often the result of high-energy trauma, associated injuries are common, and have been reported to occur in over 60% in some series (90). While both ipsi- and contralateral injuries may occur, with the foot and the tibial shaft being the most common sites, axial load may be transmitted up the limb all the way to the spine. The patient's medical history should also be carefully reviewed. Medical conditions such as smoking, diabetes, and peripheral vascular diseases are associated with poor healing and could potentially change the treatment plan.

Peripheral nerve status, pulses, and soft-tissue injuries should be carefully noted. The tibial nerve is of particular importance, as it is vulnerable in this region, and the absence of tibial nerve function is a relative indication for amputation. Significant deformity should be reduced as soon as possible to relieve tension on the soft tissues, and the leg splinted in that position. This prevents further injury to the skin, and may at times restore blood flow to a dysvascular foot. If realigning the limb fails to restore distal perfusion, then emergent revascularization is mandatory if the foot is to be salvaged. Open fractures should be sterilely dressed prior to splintage and taken emergently to the operating room for formal irrigation and debridement. Closed injuries with significant shortening of the limb should also be considered for early operation, although usually only to apply an external fixator to maintain limb length and alignment. In most cases, because of the significant soft-tissue swelling that accompanies these fractures, definitive treatment must generally wait until swelling has subsided to a degree that allows open reduction and internal fixation to be carried out safely.

Care of these fractures has been problematic. Until the 1960s, the outcome of operative care of these injuries was such that surgery was not recommended, despite the poor outcomes of nonoperative care. The first report on successful operative care was by Ruedi and Allgower (91), who in 1969 reported 74% good and excellent results among 84 pilon fractures treated operatively. However, the majority of the patients in the series had sustained relatively lower energy skiing injuries. Subsequent attempts to use these techniques on more severe, high-energy injuries led to numerous problems, with high rates of wound dehiscence, deep infection, malunion, nonunion, and posttraumatic arthritis, yielding unsatisfactory results in as many as 75% in some series (92).

Some investigators attempted to solve this problem by using a hybrid technique of limited internal fixation combined with bridging external fixation (93,94). This markedly decreased the rate of deep infection, but was associated with a high rate of minor pin track infections, as well as occasional late loss of alignment and delayed or nonunion in some cases. Limiting surgical approaches has the advantage of fewer wound complications, but often at the expense of the quality of the articular reduction. More recently, surgeons have made use of a variety of staged protocols in order to maximize the benefits of both open reduction and external fixation.

At present, most surgeons use a variety of techniques for these fractures, according to the fracture. For relatively low-energy injuries with large articular fragments, the extremity may be splinted until swelling is diminished, and a classic open reduction and internal fixation carried out. Originally described by Ruedi and Allgower, the steps are: plating the fibula, reducing and fixing the articular surface of the tibia and the metaphyseal shell, bone grafting metaphyseal defects, and then fixing the metaphysis to the tibial shaft with plate and screws (91). If patients are selected appropriately and soft-tissue problems avoided, reasonable results are typically obtained.

For more severe, closed soft-tissue injuries, a temporary external fixator is often applied to maintain the appropriate length and alignment of the limb until swelling subsides. In general, this requires one to two weeks. Mini-open reduction of the articular surface with percutaneous fixation may be carried out at the time of the initial surgery (95), or it may be done at the time of the second operation using a more conventional open technique (96). Plate fixation of the tibia is then performed using either percutaneous or traditional open technique. Modern implants, which are low profile, contoured to the shape of the distal tibia, and designed to be applied percutaneously, are useful in this regard. Some surgeons prefer to plate an uncomplicated fibula fracture at the time of the initial operation in order to assist in determining limb length and alignment; others feel that it is unnecessary to perform this acutely.

For open injuries, an emergent irrigation and debridement is carried out, followed by placement of a bridging external fixator. The patient is returned to the operating room as often as is necessary in order to obtain control of the soft tissues. If the open wounds can be closed and allowed to heal, open reduction and fixation of the articular surface can be carried out in two to three weeks, followed by percutaneous plating or by placement of a definitive external fixator. Fine-wire frames, as originally described by Ilizarov, may be employed at that time (97).

For the most severe open injuries, flap coverage of exposed bone must be obtained if an open reduction and internal fixation of the bone is to be carried out. The internal fixation may be performed at the time of flap coverage if the joint procedure can be carried out within a few days time. After the first few days, the risk of infection increases if internal fixation is carried out in a wound bed that has become colonized.

As an alternative, in a situation of severe soft tissue loss, the fracture may be fixed with a combination of screws and a fine-wire fixator. As this technique uses few permanent implants, and no bulky plates beneath the skin, it creates few wound problems and therefore results in a low infection rate. Here too, these fixators can be applied before, at, or after the time of flap coverage, or may be used without a free flap. As exposed hardware and intramedullary implants invite infection in IIIB fractures, these frames, with no permanent hardware exposed in the wound, may also be used without a free flap, with local measures such as dressing changes allowing healing by secondary intention without development of deep infection. Once all debridements are complete, the fracture may be acutely shortened to make up for bone loss (this can aid in soft-tissue coverage as well) bringing the possibility of healing without a later bone grafting procedure. The same frame can permit early weight bearing, and may be constructed to allow bone transport to make up for bone loss at the fracture site.

Ankle Fractures

Ankle fractures are mentioned here for completeness. In general, the ankle is less complicated than the tibial pilon. Fractures at this level are usually caused by rotation or by abduction or adduction rather than by axial load. Involvement of the weight-bearing articular surface is not very common. When the articular surface is involved, it is usually a small portion, and is more easily fixed than in a pilon fracture. With the exception of high-energy injuries in which the foot has been abducted or externally rotated far off to the side, they are almost always closed. When ankle fractures are open, the wound is almost always a transverse failure of the medial skin in tension. The degree of soft-tissue stripping is such that immediate definitive treatment can almost always proceed.

In the emergency department, the neurovascular status of the limb is assessed with particular attention to pulses and the status of the tibial nerve. Displaced fractures are reduced with a combination of traction and reversal of the injuring force (e.g., an injury caused by external rotation is reduced by internally rotating the foot), and a well-padded plaster splint is placed to maintain the reduction. Closed fractures that have been significantly displaced will swell significantly and should be elevated and iced until swelling has diminished to a point where skin wrinkles are present. This signals that the soft tissues are ready to accept surgical treatment.

In the case of an open fracture, the patient should go promptly to the operating room for a thorough irrigation and debridement. Unless gross contamination precludes it, one may typically proceed with immediate internal fixation. On the distal fibula, this is generally a combination of screws and a low-profile plate, although a single intramedullary screw may sometimes be sufficient. On the medial side, the medial malleolus is usually repaired with simple screw fixation. For particularly small fragments, kirschner wires may be used, and low-profile plates are employed if the fragment is particularly large. At the conclusion of the fixation, the traumatic medial wound may be loosely reapproximated if the soft tissues appear healthy, or may be closed in a delayed fashion if the soft-tissue injury is severe. In the rare case where soft-tissue coverage is inadequate, local fasciocutaneous flaps may be used for small defects and free flaps for larger ones.

Foot

Foot injuries, although often overlooked in the polytraumatized patient, are often a significant cause of morbidity (98). The foot is highly specialized to bear the weight of the body for prolonged periods and does not tolerate even small changes in alignment well. Often, after fractures of the long bones, hip, and knee have healed in a satisfactory fashion, deformity or incongruity in the foot may cause pain and impair the patient's ability to ambulate effectively.

Recently, major trauma centers have seen an increase in the volume of severe foot injuries. The combination of increased driving speeds, increased traffic volume, and safety improvements such as airbags, which protect the thoracoabdominal cavity while affording relatively less protection to the lower extremity, have resulted in increasing numbers of lower extremity injuries (99), particularly in the foot and ankle (100), where improvements in the foot compartment have lagged behind improvements in other areas.

Goals of treatment include creating relatively normal foot shape to allow use of normal footwear, obtaining sufficient dorsiflexion to permit a relatively normal gait, and establishing articular congruity and maintaining motion in the essential joints of the foot. Some articulations, such as the tibiotalar and subtalar joints, the talonavicular joint and the lesser metatarsophalangeal joints, provide motion that is essential to optimal foot function. Other joints, such as the flat joints of the midfoot, move very little and can be fused if they cannot be reconstructed, with very little compromise of foot function.

Treatment, as always, begins with the emergency department evaluation, with a careful examination of the foot for open wounds, neurovascular compromise, and immediate complications such as compartment syndrome. When the evaluation is completed, the foot should be adequately immobilized and elevated to diminish swelling. Patients with open fractures receive appropriate intravenous antibiotics and prompt surgical debridement. In the case of closed injury, the foot will often swell to a point where surgery cannot be carried out immediately. The foot is elevated until swelling has diminished—the return of skin wrinkles indicates that the soft tissues are able to tolerate operative intervention.

The techniques used for fixation of fractures throughout the foot are so varied that even a cursory discussion is difficult. We briefly consider the hind, mid, and forefoot, the essential and nonessential articulations, and the fixation techniques employed in the various anatomic areas.

Talus

The talus is almost completely covered with articular cartilage and therefore has a limited and tenuous blood supply. The superior surface of the talar body articulates with the ankle mortise, providing plantar and dorsiflexion, while the talar head and inferior facets form a subtalar joint with the proximal articular surface of the navicular and the top of the calcaneus in order to provide pronation and supination. Maintaining congruent articular surfaces and motion at both of these joints is essential to obtain optimal foot function.

The most common talar injury is a fracture through the neck caused by forced dorsiflexion of the mid- and forefoot, such as a foot on a brake during a car crash. As the energy of the injury increases, the neck fracture can become comminuted, and the talar body can be extruded from the ankle mortise, often out through the skin. Increasing axial load can result in comminution of the talar body. As a result of these injuries, the body of the talus, which receives its blood supply along the neck in a retrograde fashion, is subject to high rates of avascular necrosis in high-energy injuries. The belief that prompt restoration of talar anatomy would reduce the risk of avascular necrosis previously led to the recommendation that all such displaced injuries be treated emergently. However, recent investigations have failed to demonstrate such a benefit to emergent treatment (101). Rather, higher-energy injuries and open fractures carried the worst prognosis. Although waiting for swelling to subside in closed cases is now felt to potentially reduce soft-tissue complications, current orthopedic practice continues to advocate emergent treatment of talar body dislocations and open injuries.

Surgical exposure is generally through the traumatic wounds, or through longitudinal medial and lateral incisions. If the body is fractured, it may be exposed by osteotomizing the medial malleolus. Internal fixation is typically with screws, although minifragment plates and screws may be used to add stability when there is significant comminution (102).

Calcaneus

The calcaneus, the other bone of the hindfoot, is also injured in cases of high-energy trauma such as motor vehicle accidents and falls from a height. As is the case with most fractures, prognosis grows poorer with increasing energy of injury and with open injury (103,104), although with careful debridement and early soft-tissue coverage, acceptably low complication rates may be obtained (105,106). In order to obtain the best possible result, the surgeon must reestablish the congruence of the subtalar joint to try to prevent subtalar arthrosis, and must reestablish a normal heel shape in order to permit the use of normal footwear. In cases where the articular surface is fractured beyond repair, immediate or delayed fusion of the talocalcaneal joint may be carried out with acceptable results (107,108).

In the vast majority of cases in which internal fixation is possible, it is carried out after a period of waiting to permit soft-tissue swelling to diminish. An extensile flap is elevated from the lateral side of the calcaneus and open reduction and internal fixation carried out with screws and low-profile plates (109,110). One of the most feared complications of calcaneal surgery is necrosis of this lateral flap, which can result in a need for free flap coverage (111). In cases where the soft tissues are in poor condition and a formal approach is not possible, the fracture may be managed nonoperatively, or treated with screws or wires applied percutaneously.

Midfoot

Injuries in the midfoot are varied, as is their treatment. The midfoot consists of the navicular, the three cuneiforms, and the cuboid. Of the various articulations with the hind and forefoot, the talonavicular joint is by far the most essential in its contribution to normal foot motion and function. Motion between the navicular and the talar head, in combination with motion at the subtalar joint, provides the foot its ability to pronate and supinate, motion which is vital to a normal gait, particularly on uneven surfaces. If one articular surface of the midfoot is to be preserved, it is that of the navicular with the talus. Other common injuries include crushing of the cuboid with an axial load on the lateral side of the foot, crushing of the medial column of the foot, and dislocation of the metatarsal bases from the midfoot (Lisfranc dislocation).

In general, injuries in the midfoot are fixed with small fragment screws lagging the fracture fragments together. With fractures of the navicular, every effort should be made to restore a congruent articulation with the head of the talus. Screws lagging the navicular fragments together may be drilled into the cuneiforms to obtain additional purchase. When an axial load has been applied to either the medial or the lateral side of the foot, the medial or lateral column may be crushed and shortened. Restoring length is essential to maintaining normal foot shape and function. On either side, a small external fixator may be applied in order to bring the foot out to length. Voids left after length is restored are filled with cancellous bone graft. The external fixator may be left on as definitive fixation, or a bridge or buttress plate may be applied as an internal fixator to maintain length and alignment until healing has occurred (112). In case of a Lisfranc dislocation, the metatarsal bases are reduced to their anatomic location and temporarily fixed with either screws or kirschner wires until ligament healing has occurred.

Metatarsals

The function of the metatarsals varies according to their location. The first metatarsal is a short, stout bone that bears significant weight during the gait cycle. Displaced fractures should be restored anatomically and are generally fixed with small fragment screws or with minifragment plates and screws. The second through fourth metatarsals bear relatively less weight and can tolerate greater deformity than the first or fifth. The majority may be treated nonoperatively, although multiple or significantly displaced fractures may be internally fixed with either small plates or screws or with intramedullary kirschner wires. The fifth metatarsal is the most mobile and bears the least weight, and therefore tolerates the greatest deformity. Nonoperative treatment generally suffices. In the context of multiple displaced fractures, plate and screw or intramedullary screw fixation may be used for the fifth metatarsal.

CONCLUSIONS

The orthopedist is an important member of the team caring for the traumatized lower limb. The initial stabilization of the injured extremity, be it with traction, external fixation, or simple splints, prevents further injury to the limb during the early stages of patient care. Emergent operative interventions, such as irrigation and debridement to minimize infection risk in open fractures, and fasciotomy to relieve compartment syndrome, are crucial parts of the effort to preserve the severely traumatized limb. Although our experience with the mangled extremity is growing, we still do not have hard and fast rules as to which limbs should be amputated and which should be salvaged. Treatment must be individualized according to the characteristics of the injury, the needs of the patient, the abilities of the caregivers, and the resources available.

Once the initial evaluation and care of the limb have concluded, the orthopedic surgeon must decide how to deliver definitive care. For fractures of the femoral and tibial diaphyses, the goal is to reestablish limb axis, length, and rotation as soon as safely possible. While a variety of methods are available, this is generally accomplished with intramedullary nails. When fractures violate the joint surfaces, the goal is to restore articular congruity, if possible with enough stability to begin early motion. One must generally wait for a week or two for the swelling that accompanies periarticular injuries to diminish to a point where plate and screw fixation can be carried out safely. In severe injuries with bone and soft-tissue loss, conventional methods often prove less successful. External fixation, particularly with the techniques of Ilizarov, allows the experienced orthopedic traumatologist greater flexibility in dealing with extreme cases of bone and soft-tissue loss. In all cases, the orthopedic care rendered must be coordinated with the efforts of the general, vascular, and plastic surgeons if an optimal result is to be obtained.

REFERENCES

1. Gustilo RB, Anderson JT. Prevention of infection in the treatment of one thousand and twenty-five open fractures of long bones: retrospective and prospective analyses. J Bone Joint Surg Am 1976; 58(4):453–458.
2. Gustilo RB, Mendoza RM, Williams DN. Problems in the management of type III (severe) open fractures: a new classification of type III open fractures. J Trauma 1984; 24(8):742–746.
3. Olson SA, Finkemeier CG, Moehring HD. Open fractures. In: Bucholz RW, Heckman JD, eds. Rockwood and Green's Fractures in Adults. Philadelphia: Lippincott Williams and Wilkins, 2001:285–317.
4. Trafton PG. Tibial shaft fractures. In: Browner BD, Jupiter JB, Levine AM, Trafton PG, eds. Skeletal Trauma. 3rd ed. Philadelphia: W.B. Saunders, 2003:2131–2255.
5. Oestern HJ, Tscherne H. Pathophysiology and classification of soft tissue injuries associated with fractures. In: Tscherne H, Golzen L, eds. Fractures with Soft Tissue Injuries. Berlin: Springer-Verlag, 1994:1–9.
6. Lee J. Efficacy of cultures in the management of open fractures. Clin Orthop 1997; (339):71–75.
7. Bhandari M, Adili A, Schemitsch EH. The efficacy of low-pressure lavage with different irrigating solutions to remove adherent bacteria from bone. J Bone Joint Surg Am 2001; 83A(3):412–419.

8. Bhandari M, Schemitsch EH, Adili A, Lachowski RJ, Shaughnessy SG. High and low pressure pulsatile lavage of contaminated tibial fractures: an in vitro study of bacterial adherence and bone damage. J Orthop Trauma 1999; 13(8):526–533.
9. Bhandari M, Adili A, Lachowski RJ. High pressure pulsatile lavage of contaminated human tibiae: an in vitro study. J Orthop Trauma 1998; 12(7):479–484.
10. Dirschl DR, Duff GP, Dahners LE, Edin M, Rahn BA, Miclau T. High pressure pulsatile lavage irrigation of intraarticular fractures: effects on fracture healing. J Orthop Trauma 1998; 12(7):460–463.
11. Lee EW, Dirschl DR, Duff G, Dahners LE, Miclau T. High-pressure pulsatile lavage irrigation of fresh intraarticular fractures: effectiveness at removing particulate matter from bone. J Orthop Trauma 2002; 16(3):162–165.
12. Anglen JO. Wound irrigation in musculoskeletal injury. J Am Acad Orthop Surg 2001; 9(4):219–226.
13. Scully RE, Artz CP, Sako, Y. An evaluation of the surgeon's criteria for determining viability of muscle during debridement. Arch Surg 1956; 73:1031–1035.
14. Volkmann R. Die ischaemischem muskellamungen und kontrakturen. Zentralbl Chir 1881; 8:801.
15. Moed BR, Thorderson PK. Measurement of intracompartmental pressure: a comparison of the slit catheter, side-ported needle, and simple needle. J Bone Joint Surg Am 1993; 75(2):231–235.
16. Mubarak SJ, Owen CA, Hargens AR, Garetto LP, Akeson WH. Acute compartment syndromes: diagnosis and treatment with the aid of the wick catheter. J Bone Joint Surg Am 1978; 60(8):1091–1095.
17. Matsen FA III, Winquist RA, Krugmire, RB, Jr. Diagnosis and management of compartmental syndromes. J Bone Joint Surg Am 1980; 62(2):286–291.
18. McQueen MM, Court-Brown CM. Compartment monitoring in tibial fractures. The pressure threshold for decompression. J Bone Joint Surg Br 1996; 78(1):99–104.
19. Heppenstall RB, Sapega AA, Izant T, et al. Compartment syndrome: a quantitative study of high-energy phosphorus compounds using 31P-magnetic resonance spectroscopy. J Trauma 1989; 29(8):1113–1119.
20. Manoli A II, Weber TG. Fasciotomy of the foot: an anatomical study with special reference to release of the calcaneal compartment. Foot Ankle 1990; 10(5):267–275.
21. Lange RH, Bach AW, Hansen S, T, Jr, Johansen KH. Open tibial fractures with associated vascular injuries: prognosis for limb salvage. J Trauma 1985; 25(3):203–208.
22. Caudle RJ, Stern PJ. Severe open fractures of the tibia. J Bone Joint Surg Am 1987; 69(6):801–807.
23. Helfet DL, Howey T, Sanders R, Johansen K. Limb salvage versus amputation: preliminary results of the Mangled Extremity Severity Score. Clin Orthop 1990; (256):80–86.
24. Johansen K, Daines M, Howey T, Helfet D, Hansen S, T, Jr. Objective criteria accurately predict amputation following lower extremity trauma. J Trauma 1990; 30(5):568–572.
25. Robertson PA. Prediction of amputation after severe lower limb trauma. J Bone Joint Surg Br 1991; 73(5):816–818.
26. Durham RM, Mistry BM, Mazuski JE, Shapiro M, Jacobs D. Outcome and utility of scoring systems in the management of the mangled extremity. Am J Surg 1996; 172(5):569–573.

27. Bonanni F, Rhodes M, Lucke JF. The futility of predictive scoring of mangled lower extremities. J Trauma 1993; 34(1):99–104.
28. Bosse MJ, MacKenzie EJ, Kellam JF, et al. A prospective evaluation of the clinical utility of the lower-extremity injury-severity scores. J Bone Joint Surg Am 2001; 83-A(1):3–14.
29. Georgiadis GM, Behrens FF, Joyce MJ, Earle AS, Simmons AL. Open tibial fractures with severe soft-tissue loss. Limb salvage compared with below-the-knee amputation. J Bone Joint Surg Am 1993; 75(10):1431–1441.
30. Hertel R, Strebel N, Ganz R. Amputation versus reconstruction in traumatic defects of the leg: outcome and costs. J Orthop Trauma 1996; 10(4):223–229.
31. Bondurant FJ, Cotler HB, Buckle R, Miller-Crotchett P, Browner BD. The medical and economic impact of severely injured lower extremities. J Trauma 1988; 28(8):1270–1273.
32. Pape HC, Giannoudis P, Krettek C. The timing of fracture treatment in polytrauma patients: relevance of damage control orthopedic surgery. Am J Surg 2002; 183(6):622–629.
33. Fleischmann W, Lang E, Kinzl L. Vacuum assisted wound closure after dermatofasciotomy of the lower extremity. Unfallchirurg 1996; 99(4):283–287.
34. DeFranzo AJ, Argenta LC, Marks MW, et al. The use of vacuum-assisted closure therapy for the treatment of lower-extremity wounds with exposed bone. Plast Reconstr Surg 2001; 108(5):1184–1191.
35. Seligson D. Antibiotic-impregnated beads in orthopedic infectious problems. J Ky Med Assoc 1984; 82(1):25–29.
36. Ostermann PA, Seligson D, Henry SL. Local antibiotic therapy for severe open fractures. A review of 1085 consecutive cases. J Bone Joint Surg Br 1995; 77(1):93–97.
37. Russell GG, Henderson R, Arnett G. Primary or delayed closure for open tibial fractures. J Bone Joint Surg Br 1990; 72(1):125–128.
38. Godina M. Early microsurgical reconstruction of complex trauma of the extremities. Plast Reconstr Surg 1986; 78(3):285–292.
39. Cierny G III, Byrd HS, Jones RE. Primary versus delayed soft tissue coverage for severe open tibial fractures. A comparison of results. Clin Orthop 1983; 178:54–63.
40. Yaremchuk MJ, Brumback RJ, Manson PN, Burgess AR, Poka A, Weiland AJ. Acute and definitive management of traumatic osteocutaneous defects of the lower extremity. Plast Reconstr Surg 1987; 80(1):1–14.
41. Hertel R, Lambert SM, Muller S, Ballmer FT, Ganz R. On the timing of soft-tissue reconstruction for open fractures of the lower leg. Arch Orthop Trauma Surg 1999; 119(1–2):7–12.
42. Gopal S, Majumder S, Batchelor AG, Knight SL, De Boer P, Smith RM. Fix and flap: the radical orthopaedic and plastic treatment of severe open fractures of the tibia. J Bone Joint Surg Br 2000; 82(7):959–966.
43. Sinclair JS, McNally MA, Small JO, Yeates HA. Primary free-flap cover of open tibial fractures. Injury 1997; 28(9–10):581–587.
44. Jaffe KA, Morris SG, Sorrell RG, Gebhardt MC, Mankin HJ. Massive bone allografts for traumatic skeletal defects. South Med J 1991; 84(8):975–982.
45. Maiocchi AB, Aronson J, eds. Operative Principles of Ilizarov: Fracture Treatment, Nonunion, Osteomyelitis, Lengthening, Deformity Correction. Baltimore: Williams and Wilkins, 1991.

46. Betz AM, Hierner R, Baumgart R, et al. Primary shortening—secondary lengthening. A new treatment concept for reconstruction of extensive soft tissue and bone injuries after 3rd degree open fracture and amputation of the lower leg. Handchir Mikrochir Plast Chir 1998; 30(1):30–39.
47. Atkins RM, Sudhakar JE, Porteous AJ. Distraction osteogenesis through high energy fractures. Injury 1998; 29(7):535–537.
48. Taylor GI. The current status of free vascularized bone grafts. Clin Plast Surg 1983; 10(1):185–209.
49. Atkins RM, Madhavan P, Sudhakar J, Whitwell D. Ipsilateral vascularised fibular transport for massive defects of the tibia. J Bone Joint Surg Br 1999; 81(6):1035–1040.
50. Christian EP, Bosse MJ, Robb G. Reconstruction of large diaphyseal defects, without free fibular transfer, in Grade-IIIB tibial fractures. J Bone Joint Surg Am 1989; 71(7):994–1004.
51. Tropet Y, Garbuio P, Obert L, Jeunet L, Elias B. One-stage emergency treatment of open grade IIIB tibial shaft fractures with bone loss. Ann Plast Surg 2001; 46(2):113–119.
52. Musharrafieh R, Osmani O, Saghieh S, El-Hassan B, Atiyeh B. Microvascular composite tissue transfer for the management of type IIIB and IIIC fractures of the distal leg and compound foot fractures. J Reconstr Microsurg 1999; 15(7):501–507.
53. Browner BD, Jupiter JB, Levine AM, Trafton PG, eds. Skeletal Trauma—Basic Science, Management and Reconstruction. 3rd ed. Philadelphia: Saunders, 2003.
54. Bucholz RW, Heckman JD, Beatty JH, Kasser HR, eds. Rockwood Green and Wilkin's Fractures. 5th ed. Philadelphia: Lippincott Williams and Wilkins, 2001.
55. Taylor MT, Banerjee B, Alpar K. The epidemiology of fractured femurs and the effect of these factors on outcome. Injury 1994; 25:641–644.
56. Fakhry S, Rutledge R, Dahners L, Kessler D. Incidence, management, and outcome of femoral shaft fracture: a statewide population based analysis of 2805 adult patients in a rural state. J Trauma 1994; 37(2):255–261.
57. ten Duis HJ, Nilsten MWN, Klasen HJ, Binnendijk B. Fat embolism in patients with an isolated fracture of the femoral shaft. J Trauma 1988; 28:383–390.
58. Dencker H. Shaft fractures of the femur: a comparative study of various methods of treatment in 1,003 cases. Acta Chir Scand 1965; 130:173–184.
59. Grosse A, Christie J, Taglang G, Court-Brown C, McQueen M. Open Adult femoral shaft fracture treated by early intramedullary nailing. J Bone Joint Surg 1993; 75B(4).
60. Brumback RJ, Ellison PS, Poka A, Lakatos R, Bathon GH, Burgess AR. Intramedullary nailing of open fractures of the femoral shaft. J Bone Joint Surg 1988; 70B:812–820.
61. Kuntscher G. Practice of Intramedullary Nailing. Springfield, IL: Charles C. Thomas, 1967.
62. Brumback RJ, Uwagie-Ero S, Lakatos RP, Poka A, Bathon GH, Burgess AR. Intramedullary nailing of femoral shaft fractures. Part II: fracture-healing with static interlocking fixation. J Bone Joint Surg Am 1988; 70(10):1453–1462.
63. Winquist RA, Hansen S, T, Jr, Clawson DK. Closed intramedullary nailing of femoral fractures. A report of five hundred andtwenty cases. J Bone Joint Surg Am 1984; 66(4):529–539.
64. Mohr V, Eickhoff U, Haaker R, Klammer HL. External fixation of open femoral shaft fractures. J Trauma 1995; 38(4):648–652.

65. Broos PL, Miserez MJ, Rommens PM. The monofixator in primary stabilization of femoral shaft fractures in multiply injured patients. Injury 1992; 23:525–528.
66. Marshall PD, Saleh M, Couglas DL. Risk of deep infection with intramedullary nailing following the use of external fixators. J R Coll Surg Edinb 1991; 36:268–271.
67. Neer CS, Grantham S, Shelton M. Supracondylar fractures of the femur. J Bone Joint Surg 1967; 49A:591–613.
68. Hardy AE. The treatment of femoral fractures by early cast brace application and ambulation. J Bone Joint Surg 1983; 65A:56–65.
69. Schatzker J, Horne G, Waddell J. The Toronto experience with the fracture of the femur, 1966–72. Injury 1974; 6:113–128.
70. Giles JB, DeLee JC, Heckman JD, Keever JE. Supracondylar-intercondylar fractures of the femur treated with a supracondylar plate and lag screw. J Bone Joint Surg 1982; 64A:864–870.
71. Chiron HS, Casey P. Fractures of the distal third of the femur treated by internal fixation. Clin Orthop 1974; 100:160–170.
72. Lucas SE, Seligson D, Henry SL. Intramedullary supracondylar nailing of femoral fractures. A preliminary report of the GSH supracondylar nail. Clin Orthop 1993; (296):200–206.
73. Seifert J, Stengel D, Matthes G, Hinz P, Ekkernkamp A, Ostermann PA. Retrograde fixation of distal femoral fractures: results using a new nail system. J Orthop Trauma 2003; 17(7):488–495.
74. Schandelmaier P, Partenheimer A, Koenemann B, Grun OA, Krettek C. Distal femoral fractures and LISS stabilization. Injury 2001; 32(suppl 3):SC55–SC63.
75. Kregor PJ, Stannard JA, Zlowodzki M, Cole PA. Treatment of distal femur fractures using the less invasive stabilization system: surgical experience and early clinical results in 103 fractures. J Orthop Trauma 2004; 18(8):509–520.
76. Weight M, Collinge C. Early results of the less invasive stabilization system for mechanically unstable fractures of the distal femur (AO/OTA types A2, A3, C2, and C3). J Orthop Trauma 2004; 18(8):503–508.
77. Hutson J, J, Jr, Zych GA. Treatment of comminuted intraarticular distal femur fractures with limited internal and external tensioned wire fixation. J Orthop Trauma 2000; 14(6):405–413.
78. Arazi M, Memik R, Ogun TC, Yel M. Ilizarov external fixation for severely comminuted supracondylar and intercondylar fractures of the distal femur. J Bone Joint Surg Br 2001; 83(5):663–667.
79. Hohl M. Tibial condylar fractures. J Bone Joint Surg 1967; 49A:1455.
80. Schatzker J, McBroom R, Bruce D. The tibial plateau fracture: the Toronto experience 1968–1975. Clin Orthop 1979; 138:94–104.
81. Koval K, Helfet D. Tibial plateau fractures: evaluation and treatment. J Am Acad Orthop Surg 1995; 3(2):86–94.
82. Lindsey RW, Blair SR. Closed tibial-shaft fractures: which ones benefit from surgical treatment? J Am Acad Orthop Surg 1996; 4(1):35–43.
83. Sarmiento A, Latta L. Functional Fracture Bracing: Tibia, Humerus, and Ulna. Berlin: Springer-Verlag, 1995.
84. Sarmiento A, Sharpe FE, Ebramzedah E, Normand P, Shankwiler J. Factors influencing the outcome of closed tibial fractures treated with functional bracing. Clin Orthop 1995; 315:8–24.

85. Bone LB, Johnson KD. Treatment of tibial fractures by reaming and intramedullary nailing. J Bone Joint Surg Am 1986; 68:877–887.
86. Bostman OM. Spiral fractures of the shaft of the tibia: initial displacement and stability of reduction. J Bone Joint Surg Br 1986; 68:462–466.
87. Collins DN, Pearce CE, McAndrew MP. Successful use of reaming and intramedullary nailing of the tibia. J Orthop Trauma 1990; 4:315–322.
88. Tull F, Borrelli J. Soft-tissue injury associated with closed fractures: evaluation and management. J Am Acad Orthop Surg 2003; 11(6):431–438.
89. Sen C, Kocaoglu M, Eralp L, Gulsen M, Cinar M. Bifocal compression-distraction in the acute treatment of grade III open tibia fractures with bone and soft-tissue loss: a report of 24 cases. J Orthop Trauma 2004; 18(3):150–157.
90. Patterson MJ, Cole JD. Two-staged delayed open reduction and internal fixation of severe pilon fractures. J Orthop Trauma 1999; 13(2):85–91.
91. Ruedi T, Allgower M. Fractures of the lower end of the tibia into the ankle joint. Injury 1969; 1:92–99.
92. Teeny SM, Wiss DA. Open reduction and internal fixation of tibial plafond fractures. Variables contributing to poor results and complications. Clin Orthop Relat Res 1993; (292):108–117.
93. Pugh KJ, Wolinsky PR, McAndrew MP, Johnson KD. Tibial pilon fractures: a comparison of treatment methods. J Trauma 1999; 47(5):937–941.
94. Anglen JO. Early outcome of hybrid external fixation for fracture of the distal tibia. J Orthop Trauma 1999; 13(2):92–97.
95. Blauth M, Bastian L, Krettek C, Knop C, Evans S. Surgical options for the treatment of severe tibial pilon fractures: a study of three techniques. J Orthop Trauma 2001; 15(3):153–160.
96. Sirkin M, Sanders R, DiPasquale T, Herscovici D, Jr. A staged protocol for soft tissue management in the treatment of complex pilon fractures. J Orthop Trauma 1999; 13(2):78–84.
97. Watson JT, Moed BR, Karges DE, Cramer KE. Pilon fractures. Treatment protocol based on severity of soft tissue injury. Clin Orthop Relat Res 2000; 375:78–90.
98. Turchin DC, Schemitsch EH, McKee MD, Waddell JP. Do foot injuries significantly affect the functional outcome of multiply injured patients? J Orthop Trauma 1999; 13(1):1–4.
98. Burgess AR, Dischinger PC, O'Quinn TD, Schmidhauser CB. Lower extremity injuries in drivers of airbag-equipped automobiles: clinical and crash reconstruction correlations. J Trauma 1995; 38(4):509–516.
100. Richter M, Thermann H, Wippermann B, Otte D, Schratt HE, Tscherne H. Foot fractures in restrained front seat car occupants: a long-term study over twenty-three years. J Orthop Trauma 2001; 15(4):287–293.
101. Vallier HA, Nork SE, Barei DP, Benirschke SK, Sangeorzan BJ. Talar neck fractures: results and outcomes. J Bone Joint Surg Am 2004; 86A(8):1616–1624.
102. Fleuriau Chateau PB, Brokaw DS, Jelen BA, Scheid DK, Weber TG. Plate fixation of talar neck fractures: preliminary review of a new technique in twenty-three patients. J Orthop Trauma 2002; 16(4):213–219.
103. Berry GK, Stevens DG, Kreder HJ, McKee M, Schemitsch E, Stephen DJ. Open fractures of the calcaneus: a review of treatment and outcome. J Orthop Trauma 2004; 18(4):202–206.

104. Heier KA, Infante AF, Walling AK, Sanders RW. Open fractures of the calcaneus: soft-tissue injury determines outcome. J Bone Joint Surg Am 2003; 85A(12):2276–2282.
105. Aldridge JM III, Easley M, Nunley JA. Open calcaneal fractures: results of operative treatment. J Orthop Trauma 2004; 18(1):7–11.
106. Benirschke SK, Kramer PA. Wound healing complications in closed and open calcaneal fractures. J Orthop Trauma 2004; 18(1):1–6.
107. Huefner T, Thermann H, Geerling J, Pape HC, Pohlemann T. Primary subtalar arthrodesis of calcaneal fractures. Foot Ankle Int 2001; 22(1):9–14.
108. Csizy M, Buckley R, Tough S, et al. Displaced intra-articular calcaneal fractures: variables predicting late subtalar fusion. J Orthop Trauma 2003; 17(2):106–112.
109. Sanders R. Displaced intra-articular fractures of the calcaneus. J Bone Joint Surg Am 2000; 82(2):225–250.
110. Benirschke SK, Sangeorzan BJ. Extensive intraarticular fractures of the foot. Surgical management of calcaneal fractures. Clin Orthop 1993; (292):128–134.
111. Jachna JT, Toby EB, Horton GA. Radial forearm free flap for coverage of postoperative lateral heel wounds after open reduction and internal fixation of the calcaneus. J Foot Ankle Surg 2003; 42(5):276–281.
112. Schildhauer TA, Nork SE, Sangeorzan BJ. Temporary bridge plating of the medial column in severe midfoot injuries. J Orthop Trauma 2003; 17(7):513–520.

4

Vascular Trauma of the Lower Extremity

Fahim A. Habib

Division of Trauma and Surgical Critical Care, DeWitt Daughtry Department of Surgery, Miller School of Medicine, University of Miami, Miami, Florida, U.S.A.

Pranay Ramdev

Division of Vascular Surgery, DeWitt Daughtry Department of Surgery, Miller School of Medicine, University of Miami, Miami, Florida, U.S.A.

Darwin Eton

Miller School of Medicine, University of Miami, Miami, Florida, U.S.A.

HISTORICAL PERSPECTIVE

In the earliest of times, the prime focus in the management of vascular trauma of the lower extremity was the control of hemorrhage. Techniques to achieve this included the application of styptics, compression, cold elevation, and hot oils. Celsus described the use of ligature in 25 A.D. Galen recognized the distinction between adequacies of direct pressure for control of venous bleeding versus the need of ligation with linen for arterial injuries. Despite this, the use of ligature was largely abandoned and cautery was almost exclusively employed throughout the Middle Ages. Ambrose Paré reintroduced and firmly reestablished the use of ligatures to control bleeding from open vessels. He also developed the "bec de corbin," the precursor to the modern hemostat. The development of the stick and subsequently the elastic tourniquet allowed for elective operations on blood vessels in a relatively bloodless field.

Murphy in 1896 performed the first end-to-end anastomosis of the femoral artery for a gunshot wound to the groin. Several other advances were made in the beginning of the 20th century including the technique of triangulation to suture blood vessels and the use of vein graft. These advances allowed successful repair of the majority of arterial trauma encountered in those times.

The successes achieved in the civilian setting could not be translated to success on the battlefield. The severity of injury induced by the recently developed high-velocity explosives, slow evacuation to receive medical care, and the rampant development of infection leading to secondary hemorrhage effectively precluded arterial repair. Ligation therefore was the standard approach, more out of necessity rather than out of choice. This approach continued into the Second World War, and the dismal outcome is well reflected in the amputation rates of 49%. Advances in vascular surgical techniques, anesthesia, angiography, blood transfusions combined with rapid evacuation from the field, and understanding of the principles of debridement and delayed primary closure allowed arterial repair to be successfully applied in the Korean conflict. Of 304 arterial injuries, 269 were repaired with an amputation rate of 13%.

During the Vietnam War further advances allowed the amputation rate to remain at 13% even though the higher-velocity missiles employed resulted in a greater severity of tissue damage (1).

More recently, results are becoming available from the ongoing military conflicts in Iraq and Afghanistan. Advances in treatment applied here include the use of vacuum-assisted closure devices, liberal use of contrast angiography, and application of endovascular techniques. These advances have been offset by the increased potency of the explosives used, particularly the incendiary explosive devices. As a result, an amputation rate of 16% has been reported. Initial amputations were performed as a consequence of unsalvageable mangled extremities, while delayed amputation had an infectious basis.

These military experiences are the foundation on which the current management paradigms of civilian vascular trauma are based. With the increasing incidence of high-speed motor vehicle collisions and the epidemic proportions violent penetrating trauma have attained, practitioners that care for the injured must be thoroughly familiar with these management principles. Applications of these principles have resulted in civilian limb loss following vascular trauma of the lower extremity of about 10% (2).

EPIDEMIOLOGY

The vasculature of the lower extremity is frequently involved in both military and civilian vascular trauma. The frequency of involvement in the various armed conflicts ranges from 60% to 70%. Incidence in the civilian setting is lower than in the military setting but nevertheless remains significant, ranging from 19% to 35% (3–6). Rates are similar in the urban and rural setting (7).

The incidence is expected to increase further secondary to increases in both high-velocity blunt and penetrating trauma as well as due to the increased performance of diagnostic procedures.

There are, however, several differences between vascular injuries due to civilian and military trauma. Civilian injuries are more often due to low-velocity missiles and are associated with less soft-tissue destruction. For civilian injuries, transport times from injury to receiving medical care are short, and adequate resources for appropriate care are available. There is a higher incidence of pre-existing arterial disease in elderly victims of trauma. A major proportion of these injuries are the result of a blunt mechanism of injury, and there is an explosive increase in iatrogenic injuries due to an exponential increase in the performance of diagnostic and therapeutic vascular interventions.

While the occurrence of arterial injuries is well documented, injuries to the veins of the lower extremity are often underreported. Injured veins are often ligated and overlooked as significant injuries.

ETIOLOGY

Vascular trauma of the lower extremity may result from either blunt or penetrating trauma. Penetrating trauma more frequently results in vascular injuries, accounting for 10% to 62% of injuries, most often due to gunshot wounds and shotgun injuries. Other penetrating causes include stab wounds and lacerations with sharp objects such as glass.

Blunt trauma is becoming increasingly important as a cause of vascular injury. It accounts for 7% to 16% of vascular injuries (2,3). Certain patterns are increasingly associated with vascular injury (Table 1). These include dislocations of the knee, tibial plateau fractures, displaced bicondylar fractures, distal femoral shaft fractures, and floating joints. Blunt trauma, owing to the greater amount of force involved, results in greater limb loss (8).

Table 1 Causes of Vascular Trauma to the Lower Extremity

Penetrating
Gunshot wounds
Shotgun injuries
Stab wounds
Lacerations
Blunt
Motor vehicle collisions
Skeletal trauma
Knee dislocations
Tibial plateau fractures
Bicondylar fractures
Distal femur shaft fractures
Iatrogenic

Iatrogenic injuries are becoming more frequent as a cause of vascular injury. This is a direct result of an explosive increase in the performance of invasive diagnostic and therapeutic vascular interventions.

DIAGNOSIS

Reestablishment of circulation by effecting repair is a key factor to an optimal functional outcome and to achieve the lowest possible amputation rate.

While a high index of suspicion should be maintained in all trauma patients, certain mechanisms of injury should raise a heightened awareness. Penetrating trauma with a trajectory that passes in the proximity of a major vascular structure, certain forms of high-velocity blunt trauma, and a history of having recently undergone a vascular interventional procedure is important. The amount and character of bleeding is important in suggesting a venous injury versus an arterial injury. Also important is a history of underlying disease that may affect the vascular system, for example, coronary artery disease, diabetes, etc.

Examination of the affected extremity is performed to detect the presence of hard or soft signs of vascular injury (Table 2). Hard signs include pulsatile bleeding, an expanding pulsatile hematoma, a palpable thrill or an audible bruit, and evidence of extremity ischemia. The signs suggestive of ischemia are characterized by the six P's. These are pulselessness, pallor, pain, paralysis, parasthesia, and poikilothermia. The presence of any of these hard signs is virtually diagnostic of a vascular injury and should mandate either operative intervention or assessment by radiologic means. Imaging studies are indicated only when multiple

Table 2 Signs of Vascular Injury

Hard signs (if present, indicate the need for operative or endovascular intervention)
Pulsatile bleeding
Expanding pulsatile hematoma
Palpable thrill
Audible bruit
Evidence of extremity ischemia
Pulselessness
Pallor
Pain
Paralysis
Parasthesia
Poikilothermia
Soft signs (suggestive of possible vascular injury; indicate the need for further workup)
Neurologic injury in proximity to a vessel
Small- to moderate-sized hematoma
Unexplained hypotension
Large amount of blood loss at the scene
Injury in proximity to a vessel

levels of injuries are suspected as may occur with shotgun blasts, multiple gunshot or stab wounds, and multiple fractures.

In the absence of hard signs, other features suggestive of vascular injury, called "soft signs," should be sought because these indicate the need for further workup. Soft signs include neurologic injury involving function of a nerve in the vicinity of a major vessel, a small- to moderate-sized hematoma, unexplained hypotension in the presence of a potential mechanism, reports of a large amount of blood loss at the scene, and injury in proximity to a vessel.

A complete and thorough pulse examination of the peripheral pulses is performed. The presence, strength, and character of the femoral, popliteal, posterior tibial, and dorsalis pedis pulse must be assessed. In unilateral injuries, comparisons of the pulses in the affected extremity are made to those in the uninjured limb. Doppler evaluation of the pulses may be used if they are not palpable. The ratio of the systolic pressure in the injured limb to the systolic pressure in the contralateral extremity yields the arterial pressure index (API) (Table 3). An API of less than 0.90 has a 95% sensitivity and 97% specificity for the presence of an occult arterial injury, while an API of greater than 0.90 has a 99% negative predictive value (9). The API is therefore a useful diagnostic tool to select out patients for further evaluation. The API loses its predictive value in injuries to nonconduit vessels where significant vascular injuries may exist without abnormalities in measured values.

Plain radiographs of the involved extremity are obtained with radiopaque markers placed over each of the bullet wounds. The sum of the number of wounds and number of bullets identified must be even. If not, it suggests the possibility of bullet embolism, and a complete radiographic survey must be performed to account for the discrepancy.

Duplex ultrasonography combines two-dimensional imaging with Doppler flow and has emerged as a useful modality in the assessment of the integrity of the vasculature of the lower extremity. It may not, however, always be available, and interpretation is operator dependent. However, in experienced hands, it has a sensitivity and specificity approaching 100%.

Computed tomography is rapidly emerging as a valuable modality in the diagnosis of vascular injury involving the extremities. The recently developed four-channel multidetector technology results in a resolution that is adequate for the imaging of vessels of the lower extremity with the administration of a single dose of contrast material. This technique has the advantage of being noninvasive, less expensive, and results in less radiation exposure. It can be performed in the presence

Table 3 Arterial Pressure Index

API = Systolic pressure in injured extremity/Systolic pressure in unaffected extremity

Note: API < 0.90, suggestive of occult arterial injury: < 95%, sensitivity; < 97%, specificity.
API > 0.90, rules out arterial injury: > 99%, negative predictive value.
Abbreviation: API, arterial pressure index.
Source: From Ref. 9.

of bulky dressings and splints as may be necessary for the management of associated injuries. It is relatively operator independent and, in addition, provides information on the presence of abnormalities involving the vessel wall such as a mural thrombus. It will also demonstrate the relation of the injury to bony landmarks that allows the planning of incisions for surgical intervention. Postacquisition processing allows the vessel to be imaged in the sagittal, coronal, and oblique planes. Disadvantages include the potential for motion artifact, which may be more pronounced in trauma patients who are often poorly cooperative. It also requires the use of intravenous contrast. This limits its use in patients with marginal renal function and may precipitate renal failure if premorbid renal dysfunction exists.

Contrast arteriography remains the gold standard for the diagnosis of vascular injuries of the lower extremity. In the hemodynamically stable patient, arteriography is performed in the radiology suite. In unstable patients requiring emergent operation, an on-table arteriogram can be used to identify the presence of vascular injury.

Magnetic resonance imaging is another useful imaging technique. It often requires transporting the patient to a remote location and placement in a scanner with poor patient access for monitoring and resuscitation. Its use is therefore extremely limited in all but the most stable of trauma patients.

MANAGEMENT

Initial management follows the principles of the advanced trauma life support protocols (Table 4). Life-threatening injuries are identified and addressed. Initial hemorrhage control is best achieved by the application of direct pressure to the injured vessel. For difficult-to-visualize injuries, a Foley catheter may be inserted into the tract and inflated in an effort to tamponade the bleeding. For more distal injuries, a proximal tourniquet may be applied; however, one must remain aware of resulting ischemia from prolonged use of the tourniquet. Blind clamping of bleeding vessels may result in exacerbation of the injury or inadvertent damage

Table 4 Principles of Management

Obtain proximal and distal control
Explore the injury
Decide on damage control versus definitive management
Perform adequate debridement
Determine type of repair required
Place stay sutures to keep the arterial lumen open
Carefully pass a Fogarty catheter proximally and distally
Flush the vessel with heparinized saline
Perform repair
Flush proximally and distally prior to completing the repair
Assess the distal circulation
Evaluate the need for fasciotomy
Evaluate the adequacy of soft-tissue coverage

to adjacent structures including nerves and is never recommended. The subsequent approach is then tailored according to the location and severity of the injury and the hemodynamic stability of the patient.

NONOPERATIVE MANAGEMENT

Nonoperative management is increasingly being applied to the management of vascular trauma of the extremity because of an increased recognition and understanding of the natural history of occult injuries and the advancement and application of endovascular techniques to the management of these injuries.

Occult Injuries

In this group of injuries, despite the damage to the vessel, it remains structurally intact with flow maintained. Clinical signs of injury are therefore absent. Patterns of injury include focal segmental narrowing that may be a result of extrinsic compression, intramural hematoma, or reactive spasm. These are extremely benign and can be observed safely. Intimal flaps may deteriorate with the development of thrombosis. The later disappearance of the pulse or a fluctuating pulse deficit may indicate the presence of such an injury (10) where the pulse disappears when thrombosis occurs and reappears once the clot lyses. This occurs in 10% to 15% of cases. There are, however, no adverse sequelae when delayed repair is undertaken (11) in the group that demonstrates deterioration. Pseudoaneurysms and arteriovenous fistulae have a greater propensity to deteriorate as occurs in 20% to 40% of cases. Small lesions are usually diagnosed on arteriography or ultrasonography. Large lesions may result in an audible bruit, a palpable thrill or even high-output cardiac failure. In the presence of pulses, the API is performed. If API > 0.90, the extremity is observed. If API < 0.90, further evaluation with Doppler examination or arteriography is required.

Endovascular Interventions

Although the feasibility of endovascular techniques was described as early as 1969 (12), the use of endovascular techniques gained momentum after its use was first described for the treatment of abdominal aortic aneurysms (13). Since then it has been expanded to encompass the entire spectrum of vascular disease including trauma (14). These techniques have the distinct advantage of being able to be performed from a site remote from that of the injury. This avoids the need to operate through tissue distorted by hematoma. In this setting, it also has a higher rate of technical success and lower rate of complications because the deployment is most often performed in young, otherwise healthy, trauma patients with healthy proximal and distal segments that allow for good graft deployment. The use of this minimally invasive technique also reduces the surgical stress of an open operation that compounds the effects of the trauma.

Endovascular options include coil embolization, use of intravascular stents, and covered wall stents. The technique selected depends on the nature of the injury. Coil embolization is employed for traumatic arteriovenous fistulae and pseudoaneurysms involving nonessential vessels, e.g., the superior and inferior gluteal arteries (15,16) and the deep femoral artery (17). Covered wall stents are employed for similar injuries involving vessels essential for the perfusion of the extremity. Intravascular stents are used to treat intimal flaps. Intraluminal balloons deployed either by endovascular or open routes are used to obtain proximal and/or distal control for bleeding from difficult-to-access vessels (18). Endovascular techniques will likely enjoy a greater role as the technology improves and experience with their use increases.

PRINCIPLES OF OPERATIVE MANAGEMENT

Certain general principles can be applied to the management of vascular injuries of the lower extremity irrespective of the particular vessel injured. Prevention of exsanguinating hemorrhage during exploration of the injury is avoided by obtaining proximal and distal control of the injured vessel. Techniques that avoid damage to the vessel wall, including vessel loops or noncrushing vascular clamps, should be used. Once control has been obtained, the injury is explored and the overlying hematoma evacuated to define the extent of the injury and the proximal and distal ends of the injured segment identified. A decision for damage control versus a definitive repair must be made at this point. Factors to be taken into account include the patient's physiologic status and the trauma burden. In patients who are physiologically compromised, especially in the face of hypothermia, acidosis, and coagulopathy, or those with an excessive trauma burden including associated injuries to other structures of the extremity or significant injuries to other parts of the body, a damage control mode may be adopted. Options for damage control including placement of an intravascular shunt, ligation with extra-anatomic bypass, or ligation alone may be performed. These are discussed in detail later in the chapter. In the absence of such factors, definitive repair may be undertaken. The extent of vascular injury is assessed and an appropriate repair chosen. For injuries with partial transactions and minimal loss of tissue with an involvement of less than 30% of the circumference, a lateral repair with monofilament suture of appropriate diameter is performed. Interrupted or continuous methods of suturing may be used, however, in the latter case the potential to compromise the lumen must be recognized and avoided. In injuries with greater than 30% circumference involvement but without significant tissue loss where the injury can be resected and the ends brought together without tension, a debridement with primary anastomosis is performed. When the defect resulting from an adequate debridement precludes primary anastomosis without tension, repair using an interposition graft is performed. The preferred conduit is autologous saphenous vein, which is harvested from the contralateral uninjured extremity. Vein from the injured extremity is not recommended because it may have suffered from unrecognized injury. In the absence of autologous saphenous vein of sufficient caliber, a synthetic expanded polytetrafluoroethylene (ePTFE) graft is employed. The potential for infection due to the contaminated nature of the injuries and poor patency in below-the-knee reconstructions make it the less than ideal choice.

Once the technique of repair has been selected, Fogarty catheters are gently passed proximally and distally to clear the vessel of clot. Care must be taken to avoid overinflation of the balloon, which would result in damage to the endothelium, and subsequent failure of the repair. The vessels are then flushed with heparinized saline after which the repair is carried out. Prior to completion of the repair, the vessels are once again flushed proximally and distally, retrograde and then prograde flow is allowed, and the suture line completed.

The distal circulation is then evaluated for presence of pulses. If these are not palpable, Doppler examination is carried out. If Doppler signals are present the repair is considered complete. If neither palpable pulses nor Doppler signals are appreciated, the repair must be evaluated by direct inspection and a completion angiogram performed proximal to the repair. Any abnormality identified must be corrected. The need for a fasciotomy must then be assessed. Factors associated with an increased need for fasciotomy include an injury-to-repair interval of over four hours, the need to ligate outflow veins, and the presence of tight compartments. The adequacy of soft tissue to cover the repair is now assessed. If inadequate, transposition of adjoining muscles, use of biologic dressings such as cadaveric or porcine skin, or synthetic materials is performed. Close neurovascular surveillance in the monitored setting must be carried out postoperatively for the early detection of complications. If a fasciotomy has not been performed, frequent clinical examination and measurement of compartment pressures are necessary for an early diagnosis and prompt decompression.

SURGICAL EXPOSURES FOR VASCULAR TRAUMA OF THE LOWER EXTREMITY

The skin should be prepped down from the umbilicus to include both lower extremities. Inclusion of the lower abdomen allows for proximal control in injuries involving the femoral arteries. The contralateral extremity serves as the source for autologous vein and for interposition graft, or a source of inflow if a crossover femoral–femoral bypass is required.

Making a longitudinal incision directly over the palpable pulse exposes the common femoral artery. If the pulse cannot be appreciated, the incision is centered over the midpoint between the anterior superior iliac spine and the pubic tubercle. When the need to control the external iliac artery becomes necessary, the incision can be extended proximally and the inguinal ligament divided. Inferior extension of the incision along the course of the vessel exposes the proximal superficial femoral artery (SFA) and the profunda femoris. In this region, it is essential to identify and ligate the short, broad lateral circumflex femoral vein, because its inadvertent injury will result in troublesome hemorrhage. In the thigh, the SFA is accessed by an oblique incision made along the course of the sartorius muscle, which is then retracted medially to access the vessel because it lies in the adductor canal. Exposure of the distal-most portion of the SFA requires transection of the adductor magnus tendon.

The presence of associated injuries and need for resuscitation generally make placement of the trauma patient in the prone position difficult, precluding a posterior approach to the popliteal artery. It is therefore best accessed in this situation via a medially placed incision that extends from the posterior margin of the femur just above the knee to the posterior aspect of the tibia just below the knee. For access to the proximal portions of the popliteal artery, the medial head of the gastrocnemius and the insertions of the semimembranousus and semitendinosus are divided. Exposure of the distal portion requires detachment of the soleus from the tibia. Retraction of the popliteal vein in the lower part of the incision, which if necessary may be extended inferiorly, exposes the shank vessels. Posterior retraction of the popliteal vein exposes the origin of the anterior tibial artery while anterior retraction exposes the origin of the peroneal and the posterior tibial artery.

Exposure of the proximal portions of the anterior tibial artery is via a longitudinal incision placed on the anterolateral aspect of the calf in the middle of the anterior compartment of the leg and carried down between the extensor hallucis and extensor digitorum muscles to the interosseous membrane.

The distal anterior tibial artery is exposed through a longitudinal incision along the extensor digitorum tendon. The distal posterior tibial artery is accessed through a longitudinal incision made just posterior to the medial malleolus.

SPECIFIC CIRCUMSTANCES

Damage Control

A staged approach to the management of severe trauma is increasingly being applied when the trauma burden exceeds the patient's physiologic ability to withstand the insult (19). This approach is best decided on early in the course of the management before the patient develops the triad of death, viz., hypothermia, acidosis, and coagulopathy.

The sequence of a damage control approach includes the initial operation where the goal is to control hemorrhage, control spillage, restore blood flow if vital, and temporarily close any visceral cavity that may have been opened. This is followed by a period of aggressive resuscitation during which hypothermia is corrected, perfusion optimized, the coagulation status reestablished and hemostasis restored. Planned reoperation then follows at which time the injuries are definitively repaired and visceral cavities formally closed.

The feature unique to the use of a damage control option in the management of trauma with associated vascular injury is to distinguish between injuries that involve expendable vessels and those in which flow must be expeditiously reestablished. Damage control options for injuries involving expendable vessels include packing for muscular bleeders, balloon catheter tamponade inserted into the lumen of the vessel proximally, and if possible distally either by the open route or via endovascular techniques. For critical vessels, occlusion of which will result in limb-threatening ischemia of the extremity, use of an intraluminal shunt is the technique of choice. It allows flow to be restored without requiring the time necessary for a definitive repair. Although the flow is about half of that compared to that in the native vessel, increased oxygen extraction maintains adequate oxygen delivery to maintain viability of the tissues. Commonly available shunts such as the Javid and Pruitt–Ishihara shunt used in carotid surgery are readily available in most operating suites and can be employed. After obtaining proximal and distal control of the injured vessel, it is debrided back to healthy artery. A thrombectomy with an appropriately sized Fogarty balloon catheter is then performed. The shunt is first inserted in the distal segment. Retrograde flow is allowed after which the proximal segment is inserted. It is then secured in place using a silk ligature or a Rummel tourniquet. Development of signs of ischemia in the extremity postoperatively suggests dislodgement of the shunt or thrombosis and must be evaluated by operative intervention immediately. When extensive tissue destruction precludes the placement of a shunt, the injured vessel may be ligated. Distal circulation must then be reestablished by creation of an extra-anatomic bypass. Ringed ePTFE graft is run either from the contralateral extremity or the axillary artery to beyond the injured segment.

Combined Arterial and Skeletal Injuries

When arterial injuries of the lower extremity occur in association with injuries to the skeletal system, the incidence of limb loss is greater than with either injury alone. An isolated injury results in a 5% limb loss, while combined injuries are associated with an up to 70% limb loss.

The most important factor resulting in limb loss with combined injuries is a failure or delay in recognizing the vascular injury and restoring circulation to the ischemic extremity (20). Other contributing factors include the presence of major nerve injury, extensive soft-tissue damage, inability to cover a repair, and a failure to recognize or treat a compartment syndrome.

Hard signs of vascular involvement are less reliable in these injuries and imaging with arteriography is often required. In hemodynamically unstable patients who require emergent operative intervention, an on-table arteriogram allows adequate visualization of the vessels of the lower extremity. While Duplex ultrasonography is an alternative imaging technique, it is often difficult to perform in the presence of extensive soft-tissue damage and is often not available at short notice. Also, it requires expertise in interpretation of the images. Its utility is therefore limited in the emergent setting.

Management requires a multidisciplinary approach with care of the patient as a whole being provided by a trauma surgeon, skeletal injuries addressed by an orthopedic surgeon, soft-tissue defects dealt with by a reconstructive surgeon, and the vascular injuries managed by a vascular or trauma surgeon. The priority of reestablishment of restoration of blood flow before irreversible nerve or muscle damage ensues, usually within six hours, must be borne in mind when planning treatment.

The sequence of injury management is now well established. Concerns regarding disruption of the vascular anastomosis during skeletal repair have proven unfounded (21–23). Establishment of perfusion is therefore the prime concern. In cases where a complex repair will be time consuming, an intraluminal shunt is inserted after which skeletal stabilization is performed. In cases where the risk of infection is high, as is with the majority of these cases, external fixation is the preferred method, and then soft-tissue debridement is performed. Definitive vascular repair is then performed, and finally soft-tissue coverage of the repair is provided. A careful reassessment of the vascular status must be carried out after each stage of the repair. A completion arteriogram and prophylactic fasciotomy are routinely required. In the presence of severe contamination, use of an extra-anatomic bypass should be considered.

Venous Injuries

Venous injuries are often underappreciated and underreported. These are more common in the setting of penetrating trauma. Being more stretchable, veins are less likely to be injured in the setting of blunt trauma.

Hemorrhage of dark, nonpulsatile blood suggests the presence of a venous injury. When present, it may be initially controlled with direct pressure applied digitally or by using sponge sticks. A decision of ligation versus repair must then be made. For veins below the popliteal vein, repair is associated with poor flow rates and frequent failure. These veins are therefore best ligated. For the popliteal and femoral veins excellent flow rates and long-term patency can be achieved; these injuries are therefore best repaired (24,25). The vein can then be dissected out both proximally and distally till an adequate length is available for the placement of vascular clamps. The extent of injury is then assessed. Based on the extent of vessel wall lost, it may be primarily repaired by lateral venography, end-to-end anastomosis, or by use of a conduit. While autologous saphenous vein is the conduit of choice, when inappropriate due to size mismatch, a ringed ePTFE graft can be used. When there is moderate loss of vein wall, a patch angioplasty may be performed, and for the femoral and popliteal veins has the best flow and long-term patency rates (25). In experienced hands, the type of repair is not critical to the outcome (26). Postoperatively, the use of Dextran 40 for 24 hours reduces platelet adhesion, increasing patency.

In combined injuries involving the artery and vein, establishment of outflow by repairing the vein must be performed first. To limit the extent of limb ischemia, the artery is shunted while the vein is repaired.

Indiscriminate ligation, especially of the larger veins, results in chronic venous hypertension with limb edema, stasis dermatitis, and venous ulceration ensuing. When ligation is necessary, keep the extremity elevated, use elastic bandages to limit edema formation and the liberal use of fasciotomies.

Injuries to the Popliteal Arteries

Popliteal artery injuries are unique in their propensity to be injured following blunt trauma around the knee and the increased likelihood of limb loss with significant injuries. Their attachment to the posterior aspect of the femur and tibia by the adductor magnus and the soleus, respectively, stretches them across the posterior aspect of the knee making them prone to stretch injury. Also, even though several genicular collaterals are present, these are inadequate to maintain adequate circulation to the leg when the vessel is completely occluded. Hence, though not so anatomically, functionally it behaves as an end artery. Finally, in all but the most experienced, its surgical exposure is a technical challenge.

Improved limb salvage rates have been seen with the use of aggressive intervention (27), yet the injury-to-revascularization interval remains the most significant factor impacting outcome. Hence, delayed recognition of the vascular injury must be avoided and flow reestablished within six hours of the injury.

The approach depends on the mechanism of injury and the presence or absence of hard signs. For patients with penetrating trauma, presence of hard signs indicates the need for operative intervention. For complete occlusions with associated limb ischemia, the use of a shunt may be beneficial (28). For blunt trauma and hard signs, imaging of the vessel with angiography is performed. For patients without hard signs, irrespective of the mechanism, an evaluation for the presence of occult injury is made. This may be present in 10% to 15% and can be determined using Doppler pressure measurements and Duplex ultrasonography. The routine use of arteriography is not indicated (29).

Primary Amputation

Complete transection of the sciatic or the tibial nerve is the only absolute contraindication to limb salvage and a primary amputation is justified in these circumstances. Other relative indications that are associated with a significant incidence of limb loss include Gustilo IIIC fractures with combined open comminuted fractures and arterial injuries; threat to life for extensive hemorrhage that is difficult to control; extensive soft-tissue damage; severe contamination; and in elderly patients with multiple comorbidities (30).

COMPLICATIONS

Complications of vascular trauma of the lower extremity may result either from the injury itself or as a consequence of its management (Table 5). Further, these complications may be acute or present in a more delayed manner. Acute complications include hemorrhage, thrombosis, embolization, infection, and the development of a compartment syndrome. Delayed complications include stenosis, chronic pain, ischemic contracture, arteriovenous fistulae, pseudoaneurysms, and aneurysmal dilatation of the graft. Either of these may result in amputation of the limb, the ultimate complication of vascular injury surpassed only by death.

Hemorrhage

Acute hemorrhage is a hard sign of vascular injury. Bright red pulsatile bleeding indicates arterial injury, while nonpulsatile dark blood indicates venous

Table 5 Complications of Vascular Injuries

Acute
Hemorrhage
Thrombosis
Infection
Compartment syndrome
Chronic
Stenosis
Edema
Arteriovenous fistulae
Pseudoaneurysms
Chronic pain
Ischemic contracture
Aneurysmal dilatation of the graft

injury. Delayed hemorrhage results from breakdown of the repair, most commonly associated with infection. If the repair is in communication with the exterior, hemorrhage may ensue. Alternatively, an expanding hematoma with hemodynamic compromise may develop commensurate with the extent of blood loss. Management depends on the patient's hemodynamic stability. Unstable patents will require urgent operative intervention after measures to temporarily control the bleeding with techniques such as direct pressure, application of a tourniquet, or balloon tamponade. In stable patients, the severity of the anastomotic disruption can be assessed with imaging technologies including Duplex ultrasonography or arteriography. Additionally, endovascular techniques including coil embolization or covered stent graft placement can be employed for treatment, with surgical intervention reserved for cases that are not amenable to or fail endovascular intervention.

Thrombosis

Thrombosis is a relatively common complication and is usually a result of a technical failure. Causes include an inadequate residual lumen; inaccurate approximation of the intima; inadequate debridement of devitalized tissue; discordance between type of repair and type of injury; suture line tension; unrecognized adjacent injury; and outflow obstruction. Performance of a completion angiogram will allow many of these to be diagnosed and corrected before completion of the operative procedure. Clinically, it presents with a loss of pulses with distal ischemia of variable degree depending on the state of the collateral circulation. Immediate reoperation to correct the causative factor is required.

Infection

Traumatic injuries have a significant propensity for getting infected. The use of perioperative antibiotics, adequate debridement of devitalized tissue, removal of foreign material, and attention to nutritional support best prevent infections. In the case of extensive soft-tissue damage with significant contamination, the vessel is best ligated and perfusion reestablished with an extra-anatomic bypass through healthy tissue. It generally presents with disruption of the arterial repair with the abrupt onset of hemorrhage. Management options if infection develops include redebridement, muscle flap transposition, systemic antibiotics, and local irrigation with antibiotic solutions. Conditions predisposing to infection include primary closure of a contaminated wound, placement of the graft through an infected area, inadequate debridement of soft tissue, and inadequate debridement if the vessel should be avoided.

Stenosis

Stenosis may be acute, which is invariably a technical complication from placing too much tension on the suture line, inadequate debridement, or selection of a type of repair that is inappropriate for the extent of tissue loss. A more delayed type of stenosis results form intimal hyperplasia at the suture line that results in a reduction of the pulses. Management depends on the extent of the stenotic lesion. Resection with primary repair and resection with placement of an interposition graft are viable options. Prevention of this complication requires careful attention to detail.

Edema

Edema may result either from the increased vascular permeability that results from ischemia reperfusion injury that follows reestablishment of blood flow or from a reduction of venous outflow if the vein was ligated due to injury. Edema may result in the development or the progression of a compartment syndrome. Prophylactic or early fasciotomies may be essential to achieve limb salvage.

Arteriovenous Fistulae and Pseudoaneurysms

This is usually the result of a missed injury, where persistent wall stress at the site of weakening induced by the trauma leads to progressive weakening. It may rupture or alternatively develop a thrombus that may subsequently embolize. Diagnosis can be noninvasively established by Duplex ultrasonography or computed tomographic angiography (CTA). It is treated using endovascular or open operative techniques.

Chronic Pain

Chronic pain occurs in up to 10% of extremities following arterial injury. Exact etiology is not known; likely related to associated nerve damage (31).

Ischemic Contracture

Ischemic contracture occurs due to patchy ischemic necrosis from prolonged ischemia and failure to adequately address a compartment syndrome.

Aneurysmal Dilatation of the Graft

It is the dilatation of the vein graft that progressively occurs over time. The exact mechanism is poorly understood. The use of endovascular grafts is a tempting treatment option.

Compartment Syndrome

Compartment syndrome occurs not infrequently in the lower extremity where the muscles, nerves, and vessels are contained within unyielding fascial compartments. The ischemia from vascular injury results in endothelial injury with increased permeability that results in exudation of fluid into the interstitial space. The increased interstitial pressure compresses the capillaries inducing further ischemia and the generation of a self-propagating cycle that eventually results in tissue anoxia. Anoxia results in failure of the cell membrane Na^+/K^+ ATPase pump with a further loss of vascular integrity and worsening of compartment pressure (32). If circulation is reestablished, the delivery of oxygen to an area of previous anaerobic metabolism results in the generation of oxygen-free radicals that potentate the damage (33). Although commonly the result of arterial injury, it may in rare instances result from venous outflow occlusion either due to thrombosis or due to the need for ligation. Especially if venous ligation is combined with repair of an arterial injury, the presence of hematoma and tissue edema are also important factors in the trauma patient.

The leg has four compartments: (i) the anterior compartment containing the deep peroneal nerve and anterior tibial artery, (ii) the lateral compartment containing the superficial peroneal nerve, (iii) the superficial posterior compartment containing the sural nerve, and (iv) the deep posterior compartment containing the sural nerve and posterior tibial artery. Anterior and lateral compartments are the most frequently involved ones.

Compartments of the foot include the medial, central, and lateral compartments formed by intramuscular septa that arise from the plantar fascia. It also contains the interosseous compartment. The thigh contains the medial and lateral compartments. An often underappreciated compartment is the gluteal compartment (34), which consists of the gluteal muscles, covered by the fascia lata; it can then be further divided into the tensor, medius/minimus, and maximus compartments. It contains the sciatic nerve.

An overt or incipient compartment syndrome is frequent at the outset or develops over the course of several hours following a vascular injury to the extremity. Signs and symptoms are highly variable and may be underappreciated in the obtunded, multiply injured patient. It is therefore essential to maintain a high index of suspicion and thought of preventing it with a prophylactic fasciotomy in instances where the incidence is high. The classical presentation is with the six P's that include pain, pressure, parasthesia, paralysis, pulselessness, and pallor (35). However, in most trauma patients the signs may be masked by patient obtundation or other associated injuries and may easily be missed.

Also, pulselessness is a very late finding, with nerve damage already having occurred.

The diagnosis may be made clinically if the compartments are obviously tense. Measurement of compartment pressures using a needle connected to a pressure transducer will be necessary if the diagnosis is not as obvious. Measurement of compartment pressures is easily performed and can be done using an arterial line setup. Commercial devices are available and include ones by Stryker and the horizon pressure sense. Pressure less than 20 usually are of no consequence, while pressures of over 30 indicate the need for operative intervention. For pressures between 20 and 30, the clinical findings must be taken into consideration. It is wise to err on the side of being aggressive. Probably more important than the absolute pressure is the compartment perfusion pressure; once compartment pressures are within 30–40 mmHg of the diastolic pressure (36) performance of a fasciotomy is the judicious approach. It is important to measure the pressure in all suspicious compartments. Other monitoring techniques include the application of a pulse oximetry monitor to the limb in question. This technique has not however been found to be helpful. Near-infrared spectroscopy is another new technique that is currently under evaluation. A decrease from the normal 85% to values less than 60% is suggestive of a compartment syndrome (37).

Measurement of serum creatinine phosphokinase and myoglobin are not useful for the diagnosis of compartment syndrome. They are used to detect the development of rhabdomyolysis, which must be treated with aggressive hydration, brisk diuresis, and alkalinization of the urine.

The technique of fasciotomy depends on the portion of the lower extremity being decompressed. For the leg, a four-compartment fasciotomy through two longitudinal incisions placed on the medial and lateral aspects of the leg are used. The thigh (38) is decompressed via medial and lateral incisions. Incising the plantar fascia longitudinally decompresses the foot. The interosseous compartment must also be opened. The gluteal compartments are opened by directly incising over the affected compartment through the fascia releasing the muscles.

A prophylactic fasciotomy (39) is indicated when there has been a delay in repair of the vascular injury, combined arterial and venous injury, injuries involving the popliteal artery, severe degree of associated soft-tissue injuries, blunt mechanism of injury, associated orthopedic injuries, and the need for a massive resuscitation.

Timing of closure of the fasciotomy is based on resolution of the compartment syndrome and on the reduced likelihood of redevelopment of a compartment syndrome. Several techniques are available and include primary closure, the shoelace technique where umbilical tapes are passed through staples placed on the skin edges. Keeping the tapes under constant tension allows the edges to be brought together in a gradual manner. Several commercial devices are also available. In all there is the common principle of application of constant tension that brings the tissue back together. If the wound is very wide and cannot be brought together without creating significant tension a skin graft may be applied.

SUMMARY

The lower extremity is frequently the site of vascular injury. These may result from a multitude of mechanisms and a high index of suspicion must be maintained in all trauma patients, especially in those with suggestive skeletal injuries. Presence of hard signs generally mandates operative intervention, and use of intraoperative angiography allows for further detailed assessment in this setting. Workup in the absence of hard signs can be performed using noninvasive tests including the API, Doppler examination, Duplex ultrasonography, and CTA. Contrast angiography is being less frequently employed, but at the present time remains the gold standard. The use of endovascular techniques is increasing, and their role will evolve as technology and expertise improve. Operative interventions should follow a logical plan with care to select a repair technique in accordance with the nature of the injury. Attention to detail is key. In complex injuries with associated soft tissue and skeletal damage, a multidisciplinary approach should be used. Complications are frequent, not only from the injury itself but also from the consequences of its management. These should be aggressively sought and treated as appropriate. Application of these principles is key to management of these injuries and preventing limb loss.

REFERENCES

1. Rich NM, Hughes CW. Vietnam vascular registry: a preliminary report. Surgery 1969; 65(1):218–226.
2. Guerrero A, Gibson K, Kralovich KA, et al. Limb loss following lower extremity arterial trauma: what can be done proactively? Injury 2002; 33(9):765–769.
3. Mattox KL, Feliciano DV, Burch J, Beall AC, Jr, Jordan GL, Jr, De Bakey ME. Five thousand seven hundred sixty cardiovascular injuries in 4459 patients. Epidemiologic evolution 1958 to 1987. Ann Surg 1989; 209(6):698–705.
4. Perry MO, Thal ER, Shires GT. Management of arterial injuries. Ann Surg 1971; 173(3):403–408.
5. Dillard BM, Nelson DL, Norman HG, Jr. Review of 85 major traumatic arterial injuries. Surgery 1968; 63(3):391–395.
6. Ferguson IA, Byrd WM, McAfee DK. Experiences in the management of arterial injuries. Ann Surg 1961; 153:980–986.
7. Oller DW, Rutledge R, Clancy T, et al. Vascular injuries in a rural state: a review of 978 patients from a state trauma registry. J Trauma 1992; 32(6):740–745.
8. Rozycki GS, Tremblay LN, Feliciano DV, McClelland WB. Blunt vascular trauma in the extremity: diagnosis, management, and outcome. J Trauma 2003; 55(5): 814–824.
9. Johansen K, Lynch K, Paun M, Copass M. Non-invasive vascular tests reliably exclude occult arterial trauma in injured extremities. J Trauma 1991; 31(4):515–519.
10. Pillay WR, Pillay B, Mulaudzi TV, Mohamed GS, Robbs JV. Fluctuating pulse deficits associated with intimal arterial injury following gunshot wounds of the extremity: a sign not to be missed. S Afr J Surg 2005; 43(1):22–24.

11. Frykberg ER, Vines FS, Alexander RH. The natural history of clinically occult arterial injuries: a prospective evaluation. J Trauma 1989; 29(5):577–583.
12. Dotter CT. Transluminally-placed coilspring endarterial tube grafts. Long-term patency in canine popliteal artery. Invest Radiol 1969; 4(5):329–332.
13. Parodi JC, Palmaz JC, Barone HD. Transfemoral intraluminal graft implantation for abdominal aortic aneurysms. Ann Vasc Surg 1991; 5(6):491–499.
14. Scalea TM, Sclafani S. Interventional techniques in vascular trauma. Surg Clin North Am 2001; 81(6):1281–1297.
15. Rosa P, O'Donnell SD, Goff JM, Gillespie DL, Starnes B. Endovascular management of a peroneal artery injury due to a military fragment wound. Ann Vasc Surg 2003; 17(6):678–681.
16. Aksoy M, Taviloglu K, Yanar H, et al. Percutaneous transcatheter embolization in arterial injuries of the lower limbs. Acta Radiol 2005; 46(5):471–475.
17. Panetta TF, Hunt JP, Buechter KJ, Pottmeyer A, Batti JS. Duplex ultrasonography versus arteriography in the diagnosis of arterial injury: an experimental study. J Trauma 1992; 33(4):627–635.
18. Veith FJ, Sanchez LA, Ohki T. Technique for obtaining proximal intraluminal control when arteries are inaccessible or unclampable because of disease or calcification. J Vasc Surg 1998; 27(3):582–586.
19. Stone HH, Strom PR, Mullins RJ. Management of the major coagulopathy with onset during laparotomy. Ann Surg 1983; 197(5):532–535.
20. Cakir O, Subasi M, Erdem K, Eren N. Treatment of vascular injuries associated with limb fractures. Ann R Coll Surg Engl 2005; 87(5):348–352.
21. Howe HR, Jr, Poole GV, Jr, Hansen KJ, et al. Salvage of lower extremities following combined orthopedic and vascular trauma. A predictive salvage index. Am Surg 1987; 53(4):205–208.
22. Snyder WH III. Vascular injuries near the knee: an updated series and overview of the problem. Surgery 1982; 91(5):502–506.
23. Downs AR, MacDonald P. Popliteal artery injuries: civilian experience with sixty-three patients during a twenty-four year period (1960 through 1984). J Vasc Surg 1986; 4(1):55–62.
24. Timberlake GA, Kerstein MD. Venous injury: to repair or ligate, the dilemma revisited. Am Surg 1995; 61(2):139–145.
25. Kuralay E, Demirkilic U, Ozal E, et al. A quantitative approach to lower extremity vein repair. J Vasc Surg 2002; 36(6):1213–1218.
26. Parry NG, Feliciano DV, Burke RM, et al. Management and short-term patency of lower extremity venous injuries with various repairs. Am J Surg 2003; 186(6):631–635.
27. Thomas DD, Wilson RF, Wiencek RG. Vascular injury about the knee. Improved outcome. Am Surg 1989; 55(6):370–377.
28. Hossny A. Blunt popliteal artery injury with complete lower limb ischemia: is routine use of temporary intraluminal arterial shunt justified? J Vasc Surg 2004; 40(1):61–66.
29. Abou-Sayed H, Berger DL. Blunt lower-extremity trauma and popliteal artery injuries: revisiting the case for selective arteriography. Arch Surg 2002; 137(5):585–589.
30. Hafez HM, Woolgar J, Robbs JV. Lower extremity arterial injury: results of 550 cases and review of risk factors associated with limb loss. J Vasc Surg 2001; 33(6):1212–1219.

31. Drapanas T, Hewitt RL, Weichert RF III, Smith AD. Civilian vascular injuries: a critical appraisal of three decades of management. Ann Surg 1970; 172(3): 351–360.
32. Harris K, Walker PM, Mickle DA, et al. Metabolic response of skeletal muscle to ischemia. Am J Physiol 1986; 250(2 Pt 2):H213–H220.
33. Granger DN. Role of xanthine oxidase and granulocytes in ischemia-reperfusion injury. Am J Physiol 1988; 255(6 Pt 2):H1269–H1275.
34. Hill SL, Christie A, McDannald ER, Donato AT, Martin D. Noninvasive differentiation of carotid artery occlusion from high-grade stenosis. Am Surg 1987; 53(2):84–93.
35. Velmahos GC, Theodorou D, Demetriades D, et al. Complications and nonclosure rates of fasciotomy for trauma and related risk factors. World J Surg 1997; 21(3):247–252.
36. Har-Shai Y, Silbermann M, Reis ND, et al. Muscle microcirculatory impairment following acute compartment syndrome in the dog. Plast Reconstr Surg 1992; 89(2):283–289.
37. Giannotti G, Cohn SM, Brown M, Varela JE, McKenney MG, Wiseberg JA. Utility of near-infrared spectroscopy in the diagnosis of lower extremity compartment syndrome. J Trauma 2000; 48(3):396–399.
38. Schwartz JT, Jr, Brumback RJ, Lakatos R, Poka A, Bathon GH, Burgess AR. Acute compartment syndrome of the thigh. A spectrum of injury. J Bone Joint Surg Am 1989; 71(3):392–400.
39. Lagerstrom CF, Reed RL II, Rowlands BJ, Fischer RP. Early fasciotomy for acute clinically evident posttraumatic compartment syndrome. Am J Surg 1989; 158(1):36–39.

5

Skin, Fasciocutaneous, and Muscle Flap Anatomy

Flaps: Classification, Form, and Function

Sabrina Lahiri

Division of Plastic Surgery, Miller School of Medicine, University of Miami, Miami, Florida, U.S.A.

Rajeev Venugopal

Department of Surgery, University of the West Indies, Jamaica, West Indies

INTRODUCTION

A flap is a unit of tissue that is transferred or transplanted with intact circulation. This definition has arisen from many years of research involving the anatomy and circulation of the human body. The reconstructive surgeon possesses many options due to the vast number of techniques. This wide variety of flaps including microvascular composite tissue transfer has made possible the progression of plastic and reconstructive surgery. This knowledge of anatomy and physiology of skin and underlying structures allows the surgeon to safely and reliably restore form and function in most defects.

Over the past decades flap physiology and design have been discovered, however, recent refinements have added more versatility to flap uses. Through the use of the reconstructive ladder in combination with the vast number of flap options, the surgeon can choose the most appropriate method of reconstruction.

Any defect must be assessed carefully for structures such as exposed bone, vessels, orthopedic hardware, etc. These wounds with vital exposed structures require a durable and reliable coverage. In addition to wound healing and coverage, the aesthetics are critical to the success of any reconstructive surgery. The recipient and donor site must maintain a sense of form not deformity. Not only does form affect the outcome, but also more importantly function can alter essential daily living. Utilizing a particular muscle for coverage may cause a significant functional deficit that is worse than the original defect.

Keeping form, function, and flap availability in mind, finding the most appropriate technique can be difficult. The basic tenets of the "reconstructive ladder" should always act as a guide. The reconstruction should normally utilize this strategy from the simplest to the most complex.

When evaluating a lower extremity wound for reconstruction, the classic reconstructive ladder can be much more convoluted. The surgeon is no longer held to using the simplest first rather than the more complex. If careful planning does not start with the initial procedure, multiple procedures may end in a disastrous amputation.

Conventional reconstruction of the lower extremity has been approached by dividing the extremity into three parts. The flaps available in each third are listed and then determined which is the most appropriate for the particular defect.

In addition, there are unique characteristics of the lower extremity, which need to be considered prior to reconstruction. The lower extremity is a weight-bearing limb requiring a stable post with adequate padding and sensation. The dependent position of the lower extremity may predispose to venous thrombosis or stasis, and edema. Interestingly, there is an increase in atherosclerosis of the lower extremity arterial system which requires thorough evaluation prior to reconstruction. Nerve regeneration in the lower extremity must occur over greater lengths, which should be considered during repair or grafting. And lastly, the superficial location of the tibia can be indicative of the poorly vascularized milieu in the setting of trauma.

Trauma to the lower extremity adds yet another set of special considerations for the reconstructive surgeon. It seems that the demand for reconstruction rather than amputation has increased recently, therefore the need for more aggressive flap coverage.

Management of lower extremity wounds trails second to acute care of the critically ill patient. However, extremity blood loss and tissue contamination should be kept to a minimum prior to operative care of the extremity. Rapid neurologic and vascular assessments should be performed.

The first operative evaluation and debridement should include the reconstructive surgeon. This allows for careful determination of tissue viability and reconstructive options. Bone fixation and vascular continuity are achieved if necessary, then tissue coverage may be performed. If local or regional soft-tissue coverage is not feasible, free tissue transfer may be necessary. The timing of free tissue transfer is controversial in the literature, however, coverage within 72 hours seems to be the most commonly cited in the literature.

The complexity of lower extremity trauma can lead to multiple decision-making paths. The reconstructive surgeon must consider all aspects of the injury and the protocol for management (Table 1). These can include injuries to the

Table 1 Protocol for Management of Extremity Injuries

Assess and diagnose all injuries
Restore impaired blood circulation rapidly
Debride nonviable or contaminated tissue
Restore skeletal stability with internal or external fixation
Repair articular fractures
Repair disrupted muscle–tendon units
Repair nerve lacerations primarily if possible
Reconstruct wounds when wound is optimized
Replace lost bone
Repair or reconstruct unstable ligaments
Reconstruct lost or damaged nerve with grafts
Slowly resume use of limb, while not exceeding strength of tissues
Recognize and treat any complications

bone, joints, tendons, nerves, vessels, and soft tissue. Stability of bone and joints may depend partly on the reconstruction chosen. Without adequate blood supply or innervation the limb may prove useless.

It is of utmost importance to recognize which injuries are not amenable for reconstruction. If the patient has, for example, no sensation in the sole of the foot, severe damage to the ankle and knee, and a poorly vascularized limb an amputation may be in order. This is a controversial issue, which requires decision making between the trauma and reconstructive surgeons and family. Since the advent of prosthetic extremity, the technology has advanced considerably.

HISTORY

For many years, the design of skin flaps was based on a length to width ratio. This varied from 5:1 on the face to 1:1 on the lower extremity. This was established from anecdotal observations not scientific method. The work of Milton in 1970 (1) and Daniel's investigation of random cutaneous flaps refuted this length to width theory. It was shown that the incorporated blood supply in flap rather than the increasing width of the flap determined the length viability.

McGregor and Morgan (2) classified skin flaps as either random or axial, which promoted an increase in number and types of flaps. The rapid integration of myocutaneous flaps began with Orticochea (3), McCraw (4), and Mathes et al. (5). The early 1970s began the era of free tissue transfer. Mathes and Nahai (6) developed the classification of the vascular anatomy of muscles, which is a mainstay in the literature. Cormack (7) classified fasciocutaneous flaps according to their patterns of vascularity, thus becoming the more commonly used flaps.

Blood supply to the skin, defined as angiosomes, were pioneered by Timmons (8) and Taylor and Palmer (9). Taylor and Palmer developed the concept of the angiosome which mapped the source artery and territories to the entire body's integument.

Since the 1980s many studies have emerged with various flaps and techniques. Reconstructive surgeons are no longer restricted to skin flaps but a wide array of flaps including composite flaps. Blood supply to flaps is now the critical determinant for flap design, and the microscope has largely replaced the tubed pedicle flap. In the past two decades there has been an increased understanding of the anatomy and circulation of the human body. This has led to a dramatic increase in the number and variety of flaps available for reconstruction.

ANGIOSOMES

The intensive research of the anatomy of the soft tissue and deeper tissue vasculature has catalyzed the use of a wide variety of flaps. The concept of angiosomes described by Taylor and Palmer in 1987 (9) has elucidated the blood supply to the entire integument, deep structures including muscle, nerves, and peritoneum. The angiosome is a composite unit of skin and underlying deep tissue supplied by a

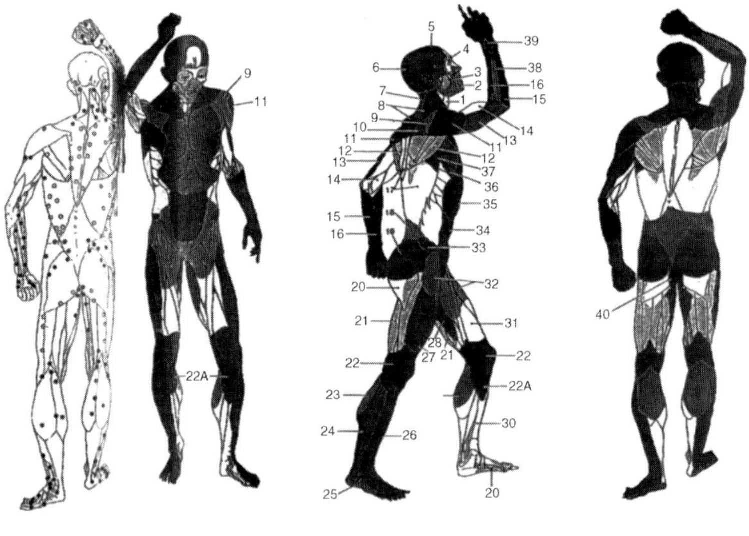

Figure 1 The angiosomes of the source arteries of the body. They are: (1) thyroid, (2) facial, (3) buccal (internal maxillary), (4) ophthalmic, (5) superficial temporal, (6) occipital, (7) deep cervical, (8) transverse cervical, (9) acromiothoracic, (10) suprascapular, (11) posterior circumflex humeral, (12) circumflex scapular, (13) profunda brachii, (14) brachial, (15) ulnar, (16) radial, (17) posterior intercostals, (18) lumbar, (19) superior gluteal, (20) inferior gluteal, (21) profunda femoris, (22) popliteal, (22a) descending geniculate (saphenous), (23) sural, (24) peroneal, (25) lateral plantar, (26) anterior tibial, (27) lateral femoral circumflex, (28) adductor (profunda), (29) medial plantar, (30) posterior tibial, (31) superficial femoral, (32) common femoral, (33) deep circumflex iliac, (34) deep inferior epigastric, (35) internal thoracic, (36) lateral thoracic, (37) thoracodorsal, (38) posterior interosseous, (39) anterior interosseous, and (40) internal pudendal. *Source*: From Ref. 10.

source artery (Fig. 1). Derived from this concept is an accurate classification of skin, fasciocutanous, and muscle flaps.

The angiosome concept has clinical applications that are important for flap design and viability. The atlas of skin flaps outlines the arterial origin, course, size, density, and interconnections of the cutaneous perforators. Therefore, it provides a template for logical flap planning and design. Cross-sectional studies conclude that the outer layer of the deep fascia should be raised with flaps in the scalp and extremities due to vessels hugging the fascia. A flap designed along the course of a cutaneous nerve such as the sural can be elevated for a long distance safely. The loose skin of the torso can be raised without the deep fascia due to the cutaneous arteries within the integument. Large cutaneous vessels emerge from the deep fascia around the perimeter of muscles and can be mapped easily.

The integument blood supply is a continuous system of linked vascular territories. The skin flap dimension survival depends on the caliber and length of the dominant vessel, the caliber and span of the adjacent captured arteries, the caliber and length of the connecting choke vessels, and adequate venous return. If arterial perforators are large and widely spaced, then the area elevated is long and wide. This is characteristic of the torso and scalp. Likewise, if the arterial perforators are close and small caliber, the territory of each is small. This is illustrated in the fixed skin of the sole of the foot. When large flaps are required for reconstruction or large vessels for microsurgery, the perforators can be chased through the intramuscular or intermuscular septa to include the source vessel. Studies show that dominant vessels course adjacent to the surface of the deep fascia. Therefore, the use of fasciocutaneous flap as a nomenclature should be carefully considered. With care the vessels can be dissected free, however, to avoid a laborious dissection the fascia is included. This dissection can also preserve the subfascial course of arteries.

Musculocutaneous flaps can be raised if the skin paddle is placed directly over the perforators of the feeding artery. In areas where the skin is tightly adherent to the underlying muscle, the blood supply to the skin is insured.

This knowledge of angiosomes provides a solid basis for transfer of composite units of skin, muscle, nerve, tendon, and bone supplied by a constant arteriovenous system. This has led to the application of free tissue transfer, in the clinical setting.

The application of the angiosome concept has been delineated for the lower extremity. The arrangement of vessels is similar to that of the upper extremity. The dominant direct perforators emerge from the deep fascia in longitudinal rows in the grooves between the muscles. The perforators converge on the convexities over the muscles. They are large and spaced apart in the proximal limb and become progressively smaller and more numerous toward the periphery.

Watterson and Taylor (11) took the angiosome concept further and revealed the venosome. In detailed study of the venous anatomy of the muscles, important anatomical observations were outlined. The venous territories in 40 muscles matched the arterial territories. Where arterial territories were linked with choke

Table 2 Classification of Flaps

Method of movement
Local flaps
Advancement
Pivot
Interpolation
Pedicle
Subcutaneous
Distant flaps
Direct
Tube
Microvascular
Blood supply
Musculocutaneous arteries
Random cutaneous
Myocutaneous
Septocutaneous arteries
Fasciocutaneous
Arterial
Composition
Cutaneous
Fasciocutaneous
Myocutaneous
Muscle
Osseocutaneous
Sensory

arteries, the venous territories were void of valves which allow bidirectional flow (oscillating zones). The muscles were classified into types A, B, and C according to the territories. Type A contains one venous territory and drains toward one end of the muscle (gastrocnemius and subscapularis). Type B contains two venous territories separated by an oscillating zone. The territories drain in opposite directions (pectoralis major, rectus abdominis, and trapezius). Type C contains multiple territories with different destinations and many oscillating zones (latissimus dorsi, deltoid, and soleus). Therefore, when a skin paddle is positioned distally on a type B or C the venous return must travel through the valves of the distal muscle prior to draining into the pedicle. In addition, Watterson and Taylor noted afferent veins entering many muscles from the superficial and deep tissues. This observation reinforces the importance of the muscle pump action for assisting venous return.

DESIGN OF FLAPS

There are numerous systems for the classification of flaps, which have evolved into three significant groups: method of movement, blood supply, and composition (Table 2). However, the most accepted classification is related to the blood

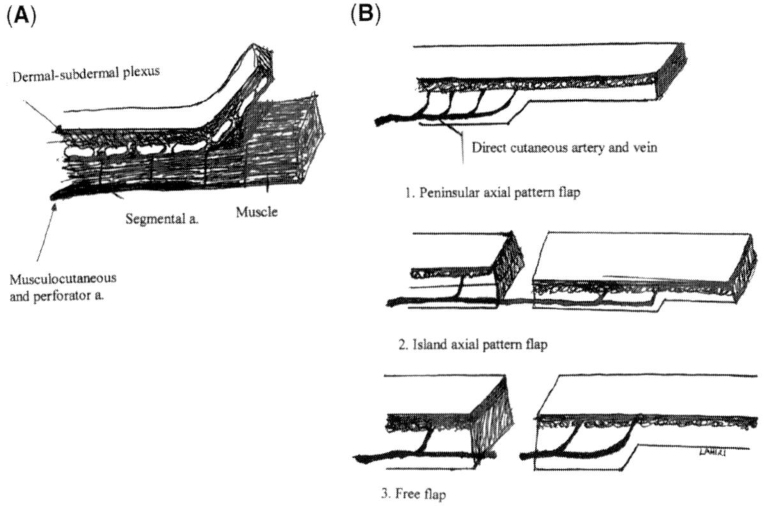

Figure 2 Earlier classification of skin flaps. (**A**) Random pattern. (**B**) Axial pattern.

supply of a flap. In 1973, McGregor and Morgan (2) made a distinction in flaps as random or axial pattern. As McGregor states, "The random flap lacks any significant bias in its vascular pattern." The axial flap contains a pedicle which has an anatomically recognized arteriovenous system (Fig. 2).

The classification of flaps based on blood supply has led to more reliable and predictable flaps. Random cutaneous flaps are characterized by their blood supply, which is not predictable but is derived from either musculocutaneous or septocutaneous vessels. These random flaps are subdivided according to the method of movement: advancement, pivot, or interpolation.

An advancement flap moves directly into a defect without lateral movement (Fig. 3). This flap can be useful when a relative skin excess is present. The typical advancement flap is rectangular and is oriented to benefit from blood supply and skin tension lines. The known septocutaneous arteries, for instance in the lower extremity, should guide the orientation and undermining.

A pivot flap can be either transposition or rotation, which derives its name from the pivot point and arc of rotation. A transposition flap is usually a rectangle or square which is located adjacent to the defect (Fig. 4). The flap should extend beyond the defect to ensure adequate flap length after transposition. A rotation flap is a semicircular flap that rotates around a pivot point (Fig. 5). The flap often must be five to eight times the width of the defect to ensure closure. An interpolation flap is harvested from a nearby but not adjacent site and is transposed either above or below an intervening skin segment (Fig. 6).

Axial or arterial flaps apply to many different tissue types such as cutaneous, fasciocutaneous, musculocutaneous, muscle, and free flaps. These flaps

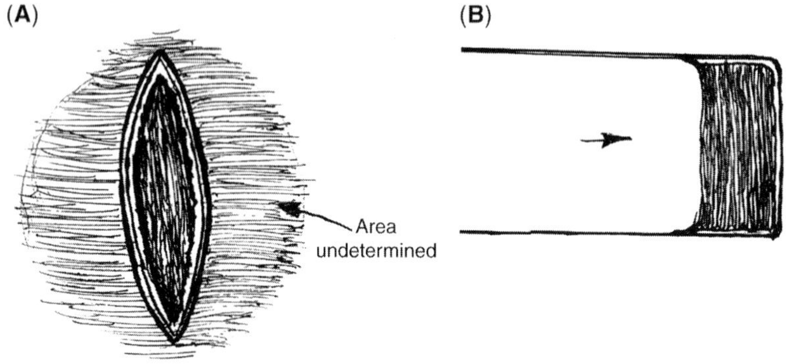

Figure 3 Advancement flap. (**A**) Simple advancement flap created by lateral undermining and straight line closure. (**B**) Straight advancement flap.

have their own classification schemes based on blood supply, which will be addressed in this chapter.

Axial cutaneous flaps include a specific artery within their pedicle and venous drainage through an associated vein or venae comitantes. Basing the flap on a specific artery allows the vascular base to be cantilevered far beyond the anatomic base. A wide spectrum of flaps exists, including the groin flap in a horizontal orientation, the scapular flap, with a perpendicular approach of the artery, and the anterior thigh flap with a perpendicular approach with short branches (Fig. 7). The dissection of these flaps requires an expert knowledge of the anatomy and skill.

A microvascular free tissue flap is defined as the transfer in one operation of a composite portion of skin and subcutaneous tissue to a distant site using microvascular surgery. This procedure is made possible by the anastomosis of an artery and vein in the flap to the artery and vein at the recipient site. In addition, other structures such as tendon, nerve, muscle, and bone can be included to add

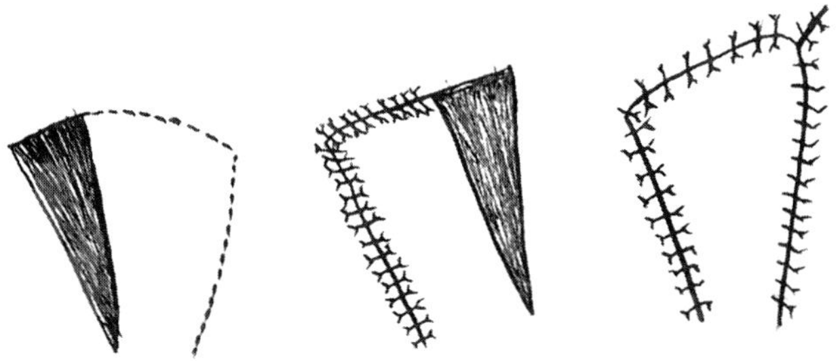

Figure 4 A standard transposition flap. Design and transposition of flap which results in donor defect. Defect closed with V-Y advancement principle.

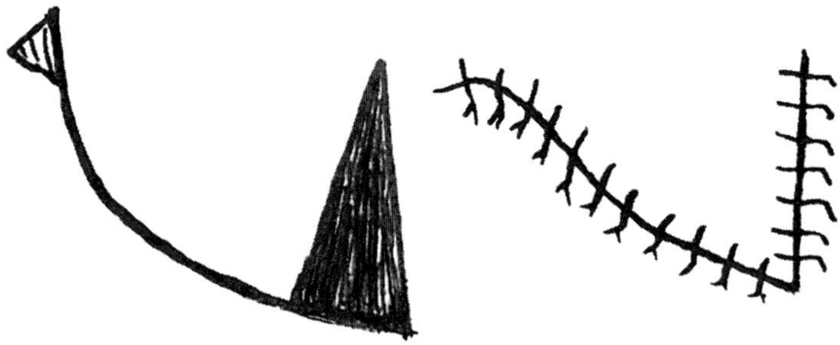

Figure 5 A simple rotation flap with Burow's triangle.

further function. Free flaps are categorized in the axial pattern flap and are subcategorized into skin, fasciocutaneous, muscle, musculocutaneous, bone, and compound flaps. The use of free tissue transfers has become increasingly important in the reconstruction of lower extremity wounds.

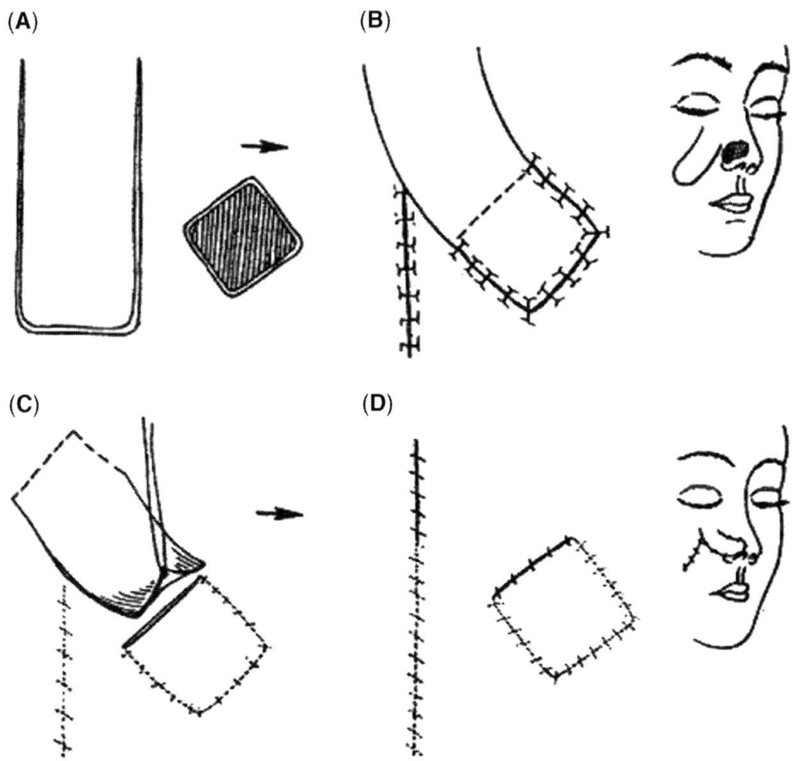

Figure 6 An interpolated flap is shown. (**A**) The flap is outlined and elevated. (**B**) The donor site is closed, and flap is inset into the defect. (**C**) Once the flap is revascularized, its pedicle is divided. (**D**) Insetting is completed.

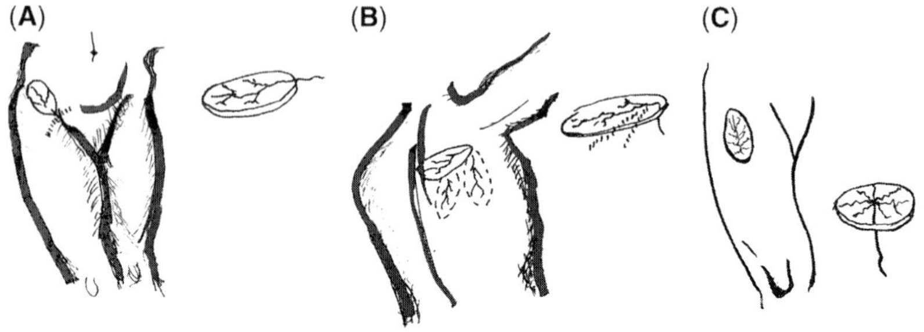

Figure 7 The vascular patterns of arterial flaps. (**A**) The horizontal approach of the vessel, as seen in the groin flap. (**B**) The perpendicular approach with long terminal branches, as seen in the scapular flap. (**C**) The perpendicular approach with short terminal branches, as seen in the anteromedical thigh flap.

FASCIA/FASCIOCUTANEOUS FLAPS

The fasciocutaneous flap as pioneered by Ponten in 1981 (12) requires the inclusion of the deep fascia to improve vascularity. Tolhurst in 1984 (13) confirmed the reliability and surgical indications for the fasciocutaneous flap. Song et al. (14) introduced the radial forearm flap, which was rapidly accepted as an island and free flap.

The vascular classification of fasciocutaneous flaps was devised by Cormack and Lamberty in 1984 (15). On the basis of detailed anatomic studies, they proposed four types of fasciocutaneous flaps (Fig. 8).

1. Type A is a pedicled flap supplied by multiple fasciocutaneous perforators at the base and oriented with the long axis of the flap.
2. Type B is based on a single sizable and consistent fasciocutaneous perforator feeding a plexus at the level of the deep fascia. This flap can be utilized as a free or pedicled flap.
3. Type C is dependent upon the fascial plexus that is supplied by multiple small perforators along its length. The perforators reach it from a deep artery by passing along the fascial septum between muscles. It is used as a free flap by taking the skin, fascia, and vascular pedicle. The radial forearm flap is a typical example.
4. Type D is an osteomusculofasciocutaneous free flap. An extension of C, the fascial septum is taken with adjacent muscle and bone.

Fasciocutaneous flaps of the upper or lower extremity have many advantages. The flaps are frequently simple to elevate, less bulky, highly reliable, and with little functional impairment. The fasciocutaneous flap is less resistant to infection and may not be a good choice for exposed hardware and chronically infected wounds.

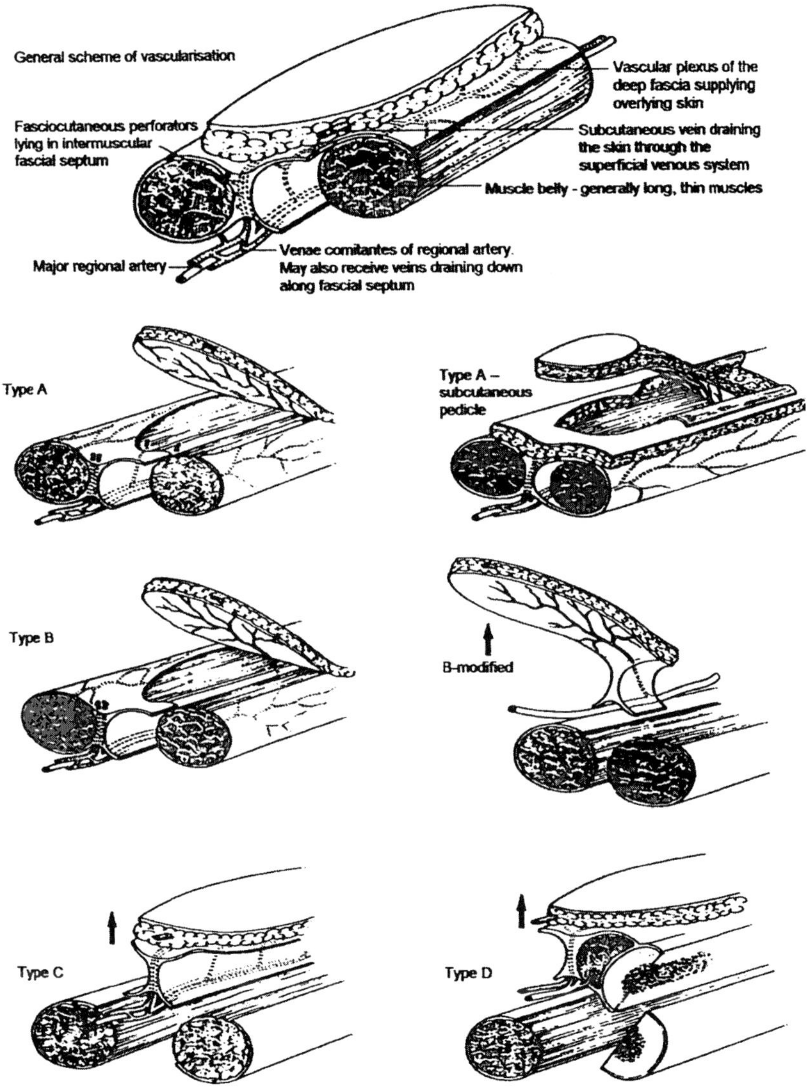

Figure 8 A classification of fasciocutaneous flaps. *Source*: From Ref. 16.

MUSCLE/MUSCULOCUTANEOUS FLAPS

The initial work describing the anatomy, principles, and clinical applications of the muscle flap was done by Ger from 1966 to 1972 (17). His work led to the classification and widespread use in plastic surgery.

Musculocutaneous flaps were first used clinically by Owens in 1955 (18). This clinical experience has been furthered by McGraw, Orticochea, Mathes, and

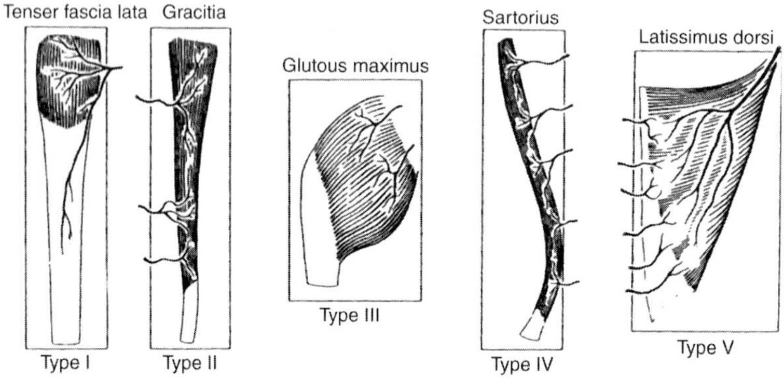

Figure 9 Patterns of vascular anatomy of muscle: type I, one vascular pedicle; type II, dominant pedicle(s) plus minor pedicles; type III, two dominant pedicles; type IV, segmental vascular pedicles; type V, dominant pedicle plus secondary segmental pedicles. *Source*: From Ref. 19.

Nahai. This versatile flap was initially perceived as a composite flap of muscle, subcutaneous tissue, and skin, which could replace the muscle flap and skin graft. However, the use of both muscle and myocutaneous flaps has been equivalent.

The classification of muscle circulation is based on the vascular pedicle or pedicles that enters the muscle belly between its origin and insertion. If more than one vascular pedicle enters a muscle, the larger pedicle generally enters the portion of muscle located at the proximal end of an extremity or midline of the trunk. In 1981, Mathes and Nahai (6) devised a classification of muscle flaps which has become the standard. The classification describes five patterns of circulation from the anatomic studies (Fig. 9).

1. Type I muscles include one vascular pedicle. Muscles in this group include the gastrocnemius, rectus femoris, and tensor fascia lata.
2. Type II muscles demonstrate one or more large vascular pedicles entering in close proximity to the muscle origin or insertion and small vascular pedicles entering the muscle belly. Muscles in this group include the soleus, vastus medialis, biceps femoris, semitendinosis, and trapezius. This is the most common pattern observed in the anatomical studies of the human body.
3. Type III muscles include two large vascular pedicles, each arising from a separate regional artery. Muscles in this group include the gluteus maximus, rectus abdominus, serratus anterior, and semimembranosus.
4. Type IV muscles demonstrate multiple pedicles entering the muscle between its origin and insertion. These pedicles are similar in size and have a segmental distribution. This group includes the sartorius, flexor hallucis longus, and extensor digitorum longus.

5. Type V muscles include a single large vascular pedicle close to the muscle insertion and segmental pedicles entering the muscle close to its origin. The pectoralis major and latissimus dorsi muscles are examples of this type.

The initial work with the myocutaneous flaps involved the closure of difficult wounds in which the muscle was used to support the essential cutaneous flap. Additional clinical experience has demonstrated that the muscle provides bulk for filling dead space, and the high vascularity helps to control infection. It is critical to design the flap overlying the musculocutaneous arteries emerging from the underlying muscle. In 1981, Mathes and Chang (19) studied the effects of bacterial inoculation in musculocutaneous and random-pattern flaps. Compared to random flaps musculocutaneous flaps recovered rapidly to the bacterial challenge without necrosis and decreased the bacterial count in wound spaces.

The surgeon must compare and contrast muscle flaps with myocutaneous flaps for reconstruction of a defect. When an aesthetic skin matches or a substantial amount of soft tissue is necessary, as is often the case for breast reconstruction, a myocutaneous flap is the first choice. In other areas, such as the lower extremity, the myocutaneous flap offers more size; however, the donor site is often unacceptable. Utilizing a muscle flap is a desirable option for lower extremity reconstruction due to improved donor site appearance. In 1977, Ger (20) reported some of the original experiences with muscle flaps for lower extremity reconstruction. He studied patients with delayed closure, secondary closure after initial failure, and chronic osteomyelitis. With the use of muscle flaps and skin grafting, all wounds healed completely. The durability of the muscle flap with a skin graft has been shown to be very effective in the literature and does not justify the selection of the musculocutaneous flap. In the lower extremity, the muscle flap has replaced the musculocutaneous flap for both local and free flap reconstruction.

The selection of a muscle flap should meet specific criteria: (i) accessible, (ii) limitation of functional loss, (iii) adequate muscle size, (iv) easily transposed into wound, and (v) reliable vascular pedicle.

BONE VASCULAR CLASSIFICATION

Bone is vascularized through periosteal and endosteal sources. The blood supply of bone is complex and based on nutrient vessels. These vessels enter the bone directly and through connections between muscles and bone. Bone and osteocutaneous flaps are used in free tissue transfers. The most commonly transferred bones include the fibula, iliac crest, scapula, and the radius.

The classification of bone flaps varies with each flap. The pattern of circulation to the scapula and radius is classified by the parent flap as these bones are transposed as a part of the parent flap. The fibula and iliac crest are often transferred as bone only flaps. The iliac crest is classified as a type I from direct vessels off the deep circumflex iliac artery. The fibula is classified as type V as a result of the dominant nutrient pedicle from the peroneal artery and segmental periosteal pedicles. This type of circulation allows for multiple osteotomies.

MICROVASCULAR COMPOSITE TISSUE TRANSPLANTATION

Microvascular surgery evolved from the progression of surgical technique, the operating microscope, microinstruments, and sutures. In 1960, Jacobson et al. (21) reported microsurgical anatomosis in animal arteries 1.4 mm. Nakayama et al. reported the first clinical series of free tissue microsurgical transfers in 1964 (22). Komatsu and Tamai performed the first successful replantation of an amputated digit using the microscope in 1968 (23). In 1971, Antia and Buch (24) reported a superficial epigastric artery free flap to the face of a patient some years prior. Anastomosis of vessels with diameters of 0.5 – 2 mm became possible with a high patency rate. Because flaps are based on reliable pedicles, transplantation to a distant site is a viable option due to the anastomosis of an artery and vein. This enables the surgeon to transfer flaps based on suitability for defect coverage rather than proximity. Free flap reconstruction has become an important option for lower extremity defects, particularly the distal leg.

REFERENCES

1. Milton SH. Pedicled skin-flaps: the fallacy of the length-width ratio. Br J Sur 1970; 57:502.
2. McGregor IA, Morgan G. Axial and random pattern flaps. Br J Plast Surg 1973; 26:202.
3. Orticochea M. The musculo-cutaneous flap method: an immediate and heroic substitute for the method of delay. Br J Plast Surg 1972; 25:106.
4. McCraw JB, Dibbell DG, Carraway JH. Clinical definition of independent myocutaneous vascular territories. Plast Reconstr Surg 1977; 60(3):341.
5. Mathes SJ, Vasconez LO, Jurkiewicz MJ. Extensions and further applications of muscle flap transposition. Plast Reconstr Surg 1977; 60(1):6.
6. Mathes SJ, Nahai F. Classification of the vascular anatomy of muscles: experimental and clinical correlation. Plast Reconstruct Surg 1981; 67(2):177.
7. Cormack GC, Lamberty BG. A classification of fascio-cutaneous flaps according to their patterns of vascularisation. Br J Plast Surg 1984; 37:80.
8. Timmons MJ. Landmarks in the anatomical study of the blood supply of the skin. Br J Plast Surg 1985; 38:197.
9. Taylor GI, Palmer JH. The vascular territories (angiosomes) of the body: experimental study and clinical applications. Br J Plast Surg 1987; 40:113.
10. Taylor GI, Palmer JH. The vascular territories (angiosomes) of the body: experimental study and clinical applications. Br J Plast Surg 1987; 40:131.
11. Watterson PA, Taylor GI, Crock JG. The venous territories of muscles: anatomical study and clinical implications. Br J Plast Surg 1988; 41:569.
12. Ponten B. The fasciocutaneous flap: its use in soft tissue defects of the lower leg. Br J Plast Surg 1981; 34:215.

13. Tolhurst DE. Surgical indications for fasciocutaneous flaps. Ann Plast Surg 1984; 13(6):495.
14. Song YG, Chen GZ, Song YL. The free thigh flap: a new free flap concept based on the septocutaneous artery. Br J Plast Surg 1984; 37:149.
15. Cormack GC, Lamberty BGH. A classification of fascio-cutaneous flaps according to their patterns of vascularisation. Br J Plast Surg 1984; 37:80.
16. Cormack GC, Lamberty BGH: The Arterial Anatomy of Skin Flaps. Edinburgh, Churchill Livingstone, 1986.
17. Ger R. Current Problems in Surgery. Chicago, Year Book Medical Publishers, 1972:3.
18. Owens N. A compound neck pedicle designed for the repair of massive facial defects. Plast Reconstr Surg 1955; 15:369.
19. Chang N, Mathes SJ. Comparison of the effect of bacterial inoculation in musculocutaneous and random-pattern flaps. Plast Reconstr Surg 1982; 70(1):1.
20. Ger R. Muscle transposition for treatment and prevention of chronic post-traumatic osteomyelitis of the tibia. J Bone Joint Surg 1977; 59A:784.
21. Jacobson JH, Suarez EL. Microsurgery in anastomosis of small vessels. Surg Forum 1960; 11:243.
22. Nakayama K et al. Experience with free autografts of the bowel with a new venous anastomosis apparatus. Surgery 1964; 55:796.
23. Tamai S. Digital replantation. Clin Plast Surg 1978; 5:195.
24. Antia NH, Buch VI. Transfer of an abdominal dermo-fat graft by direct anastomosis of blood vessels. Br J Plast Surg 1971; 24:15.

6

Soft-Tissue Repair for Proximal and Middle Third Problems

Joshua Kreithen
Division of Plastic Surgery, University of Florida School of Medicine, Gainesville, Florida, U.S.A.

Kerri Woodberry
Division of Plastic Surgery, Saint Louis University School of Medicine, St. Louis, Missouri, U.S.A.

Seung-Jun O
Division of Plastic Surgery, Medical University of South Carolina, Charleston, South Carolina, U.S.A.

INTRODUCTION

Soft-tissue reconstruction of the lower extremity following trauma can be extremely challenging and complex. Severe lower extremity trauma often causes damage to the soft tissue and bones with or without underlying nerve, muscle, and tendon injuries. The management of these injuries involves a collaborative effort between the orthopedic surgeon, trauma surgeon, plastic surgeon, and vascular surgeon. The final outcome should render a pain-free lower extremity that is both functional and aesthetically acceptable.

The purpose of this chapter is to discuss the management of soft-tissue injuries of the lower extremity with particular emphasis on reconstruction in the upper and middle third leg wounds. Reconstructive options are influenced by a variety of factors including: (i) the size and location of the soft-tissue defect, (ii) the mechanism of injury, (iii) the presence of injury to surrounding structures, and (iv) the cosmetic and functional expectations of the patient. In addition, the general medical condition of the patient as well as associated traumatic injuries must be identified and addressed. The reconstructive ladder is a guide when approaching these lower extremity wounds. Wound coverage can be achieved with primary or secondary closure, skin grafting, local flap reconstruction, distant flap reconstruction, and/or free tissue transfer. Although microvascular reconstruction of the lower extremity has become popular, pedicled flap reconstruction continues to play a pivotal role in reconstruction of the upper and middle third lower extremity defects.

HISTORY

The management of lower extremity wounds has evolved through the years and has been profoundly influenced by the experiences gained during the times of war. Fundamental concepts such as adequate wound debridement and skeletal stabilization have developed during the World Wars and the Korean War. Introduction of antibiotics and improvements with anesthetic techniques further improved the outcomes of lower extremity wounds. Surgical advances such as microvascular free tissue transfer and distraction osteogenesis have added to the armamentarium for the treatment of complex lower extremity wounds.

WOUND DEBRIDEMENT

In the management of lower extremity trauma, it is important to recognize the mechanism of the injury and determine whether the wound is caused by high- or low-energy impact. Gustilo classified open fractures based on soft-tissue injury. Grade I wounds have less than 1 cm defect. Grade II fractures have wounds, greater than 1 cm, without extensive soft-tissue disruption. Grade IIIA wounds have extensive soft-tissue disruption with adequate coverage of bone. Grade IIIB wounds have extensive soft-tissue involvement with periosteal stripping, exposed bone, and undermining of the wound. Grades IIIC are associated with arterial injury requiring repair.

A key concept of soft-tissue reconstruction of the lower extremity is to ensure adequate debridement and irrigation of the wound. Wounds are treated with initial debridement and bone stabilization by the orthopedic surgeons. Serial debridement is then done every few days until devitalized tissue has been removed with no evidence of infection or necrosis. The endpoint of wound debridements should be a clean, healthy wound bed with healthy, bleeding tissue. The use of fluorescein can be a useful adjunct to determine tissue viability, especially the skin. Wound cultures at the time of debridement can be useful to direct culture-specific antibiotic therapy. Empiric broad-spectrum antibiotics may be used when dealing with an obviously infected or grossly contaminated wound. A combination of surgical debridement and appropriate antibiotic coverage will help prepare the wound for later coverage.

TIMING

The ideal time for soft-tissue reconstruction in lower extremity trauma is somewhat controversial. It often depends on the severity of the injury, the mechanism of the injury, and the medical status of the patient. Godina proposed early closure of the wound within 72 hours. Decreased flap failure, decreased risk of infections, improved bone healing, fewer numbers of operations, and shorter length of stay for patients were observed. According to Yaremchuk, stabilization of the bone with adequate debridement is the most important first step. Afterwards, serial debridement, soft-tissue coverage, and delayed bone reconstruction is the recommended global treatment plan. Francel showed that the results of lower extremity reconstruction are the same with delayed soft-tissue closure versus early closure. Typically, the timing of reconstruction is divided into the acute phase (within 72 hours), the subacute phase (between one and three weeks), and the chronic phase (after three weeks). Obviously, timing is also dependent on the patient's other life-threatening injuries and requirements for treatment of other problems.

VASCULAR INJURIES

In assessing patients for soft-tissue reconstruction, it is important to determine the vascular status of the lower extremity. Clinical exam, including observation of the color of the extremity, the presence of capillary refill, assessment of the lower extremity pulses, and tissue turgor, should be preformed. The Doppler ultrasound can be a useful adjunct to the clinical exam to help determine the pulse status of the extremity. Occasionally, angiography is needed, particularly in the setting of massive lower extremity trauma and/or an ischemic lower extremity. Dublin reported that angiography may not be necessary prior to microvascular reconstruction in patients with adequate pulses that are demonstrated on examination. However, angiography is utilized when the status of recipient vessels for microvascular reconstruction cannot be determined by clinical exam.

In the event of a popliteal vessel injury, the patient needs emergent repair or reconstruction of the vessel. Popliteal vessel injuries are often associated with three posterior dislocations. Vascular injuries distal to the trifurcation are treated based on the patency of the other vessels. If all vessels are injured, then at least one of the vessels needs to be repaired or reconstructed. If there is only one vessel injury, then ligation is a reasonable option for treatment. If two vessels are injured, some would recommend repair of at least one of the vessels; however, there is no study to prove that two-vessel potency is any better than one vessel in the lower extremity.

NERVE INJURIES

Although nerve injuries can be repaired, overall the results are not very good. Significant nerve injury with an insensate foot may be an indication for primary amputation. If the peroneal nerve is injured, the patient will have a foot drop with loss of sensation along the dorsal aspect of the foot. Without peroneal nerve repair, function can be restored with tendon transfers. If the posterior tibial nerve is injured, the most devastating functional loss is the absence of plantar sensation.

The patient will also have loss of plantar flexion and difficulty with step off and ambulation. Primary repair of posterior tibial nerve injuries can be undertaken or can be reconstructed with nerve graft.

The results are dependent on age of the patient, the level of injury, the amount of damage to surrounding tissue, and the nerve gap. Complex orientation of the fascicles in lower extremity nerves often leads to poor results. Also, the greater the distance from the motor endplates, the greater the chances of end organ atrophy. Despite the seemingly poor results of nerve repair for lower extremity trauma, there have been reports of good results, particularly in children. In the event that the patient has a nerve or vascular injury, soft-tissue reconstruction may be required for coverage of exposed nerves or vessels immediately. In the face of a contaminated wound, it is best to delay nerve repair until the wound has been adequately debrided.

PRIMARY CLOSURE

Occasionally in the lower extremity, wounds can be closed primarily after adequate debridement. Most of these are lower-grade injuries without a significant surrounding zone of injury. With severe trauma it is often difficult to determine the zone of injury. The patient may have ongoing tissue loss that is not readily identifiable. In this case, delayed primary closure following multiple serial debridements is indicated. With significant high-velocity trauma, such as seen following motor vehicle accidents and gunshot wounds, the patient can have a large zone of devitalized tissue. Another consideration in planning closure of the skin is the presence of fracture blisters. Fracture blistering can occur secondary to soft-tissue swelling; with an increased pressure in the dermis there is an exudate of fluid, which results in blisters. They are usually small and located often in areas of minimal subcutaneous tissue such as the ankle. Incisions through the area of fracture blistering can result in increased risk of wound infection.

SKIN GRAFTS

Skin grafts are often used for reconstruction in the lower extremity if delayed primary closure is not feasible. Skin grafts can be split or full thickness. They can be meshed or nonmeshed. The nonmeshed skin grafts tend to be more cosmetically acceptable. However, meshed skin grafts can be expanded to increase the amount of available skin. Skin grafts require a vascularized bed and can be placed on subcutaneous tissue, muscle, paratenon, or periosteum. They can occasionally be placed over neurovascular bundles, however, it is preferred that nerves and vessels have better coverage with muscle or fascial flaps. There are reports of successful skin grafts taken directly on limited decorticated bone after a period of healing, allowing for granulation tissue formation. This option is rarely used today and is presented for historical purposes only.

LOCAL FLAPS

As we ascend the reconstructive ladder in determining options for lower extremity reconstruction, local flaps can be used particularly for small defects. Initially flaps were based on random blood supply and therefore limited by the one-to-one ration. Random flaps in the lower extremity have more recently been replaced by the increasing use of fasciocutaneous flaps for lower extremity reconstruction. Axial flaps, which have their own blood supply, are preferred for lower extremity reconstruction and have a longer length-to-width ratio.

FASCIOCUTANEOUS FLAPS

Fasciocutaneous flaps contain skin, subcutaneous tissue, and deep fascia. Because the muscle is usually preserved, the function of the lower extremity is not affected. These flaps are typically designed in the lower extremity based on the perforators of the anterior tibial, posterior tibial, and peroneal vessels. Knowledge and familiarity of the vascular anatomy is critical to the successful design and execution of the flap. Ponten described the most commonly used flap based on perforators of the posterior tibial vessel. In addition, Amarante described a distally based flap over the posterior tibial vessels. Because of the critical reliance on muscular and septocutaneous perforators, these flaps can be unreliable in the setting of severe lower extremity trauma with a significant zone of injury. Fasciocutaneous flaps can be deepithelialized to create just a subcutaneous and fascial component. They can be contoured to fill soft-tissue defects. They are simple to design and there is minimal functional loss associated with them.

Fasciocutaneous flaps are often used when a patient's medical problems preclude free tissue transfer, or when there is significant muscle damage precluding muscle use. Fasciocutaneous flaps may be used for reconstruction primarily or as a secondary procedure following failure of free tissue transfer or a muscle flap. Unfortunately, fasciocutaneous flaps are not ideal for elderly patients, particularly those with atherosclerotic disease, diabetes, or vascular insufficiency, or any patient with significant high-energy wounds. Following harvest, the donor site needs to be skin graded. The saphenous flap has been described for reconstruction around the anterior knee and proximal tibia.

DISTANT FLAPS

The cross-leg flap is mentioned for historical purposes since it is rarely used now with the increased use of free tissue transfer. However, cross-leg flaps can be used in children because they can tolerate the period of immobilization better. Caution must be executed in the use of cross-leg flaps in adults because of the risk of contractures and deep vein thrombosis. There have been recent reports on the use of free tissue transfer in the contralateral extremity following trauma in cases where there is not an adequate recipient vessel. Later the free tissue transfer is used as a cross-leg flap for reconstruction of the traumatic defect.

MUSCLE FLAPS

The mainstay of reconstruction of proximal and middle third defects of the lower extremity has been reconstruction with muscle flaps. Muscle flaps have been shown to be more resistant to infection. Mathes and Nahai classified muscle flaps based on vascularity. It is important to know the vascular anatomy in order to adequately design and raise muscle flaps. Type I flaps have one dominant vascular pedicle. Type II flaps have one dominant pedicle and a secondary minor pedicle. Type III flaps have two dominant pedicles. Type IV flaps have segmental pedicles, and type V flaps have one dominant pedicle and a secondary dominant segmental blood supply. In addition to the muscle components, skin can be included in these flaps based on perforators.

UPPER THIRD RECONSTRUCTION

Gastrocnemius

When discussing lower extremity reconstruction, the leg is divided into upper, middle, and lower thirds. The primary muscle flap used for reconstruction of the upper third is the gastrocnemius flap. The gastrocnemius flap can be used for coverage around the knee joint, proximal tibia, and popliteal fossa. The muscle can extend to 10 cm above the knee. The medial gastrocnemius, lateral gastrocnemius, or both can be harvested. Most commonly the medial gastrocnemius is used because it is larger. The lateral gastrocnemius does not reach along the medial leg. Harvest of the gastrocnemius flap, particularly if taken with skin, can leave a significant donor defect. The gastrocnemius functions in plantar flexion, and it can be sacrificed if the soleus muscle is intact. From a functional standpoint, gastrocnemius harvest can affect running, and therefore should be used cautiously in athletes.

In the anatomy of the gastrocnemius the blood supply is based on medial and lateral branches of the sural artery, which is a branch of the popliteal artery. It enters the muscle proximally and, therefore, this is a Mathes and Nahai type I muscle flap with proximal dominant blood supply. The gastrocnemius can be extended with a fasciocutaneous component and therefore can reach as high as 15 cm above the knee or 10 cm above the ankle. If there is concern for the flap to survive an extended reach, the flap may need to be delayed by incising around the edges of the skin prior to the harvest.

The gastrocnemius is the largest and most superficial muscle in the superficial posterior compartment of the leg. The origin is off the lateral and medial femoral condyles, and it inserts into the calcaneus through the Achilles tendon. It is superficial to the soleus with the plantaris tendon noted to run between the two muscles. A tibial nerve branch for the motor component innervates the gastrocnemius muscle, and the sural and saphenous nerves provide the sensory component.

In harvesting the medial gastrocnemius, an incision is made from the medial tibial condyle to within 10 cm above the ankle. The muscle is separated from the soleus muscle, dissected, and divided at the posterior midline raphe. It is important to watch for the sural nerve during this dissection as it runs between the medial and lateral heads of the gastrocnemius. The gastrocnemius flap can be divided at its origin on the femoral condyles in essence creating an island flap, which can increase its arc of rotation and add an additional 5 cm of length.

The lateral gastrocnemius harvest begins with an incision 2 cm posterior to and parallel to the fibula. The peroneal nerve wraps around the fibular neck and should be identified early in the dissection in order to avoid injury to the peroneal nerve. The myocutaneous component of the lateral gastrocnemius flap extends to within 10 cm from the lateral malleolus. The lateral head of the gastrocnemius is about 3–4 cm shorter than the medial head.

FASCIOCUTANEOUS FLAPS

Saphenous Flap

The saphenous flap, a facsciocutaneous flap, is located on the medial aspect of the knee and upper medial calf. The maximal area of tissue that can be transferred is approximately 7×20 cm^2. The standard design is a U-shaped flap with the apex inferior to the medial knee. This flap can be transposed to the anterior knee. A reverse flap with the apex above the knee can be transposed to cover the proximal calf or an amputation stump.

The dominant pedicle is the saphenous branch of the descending genicular artery that is a branch of the superficial femoral artery. Fasciocutaneous branches course around the sartorius and supply the skin and may have dominant perforators anterior or posterior to the muscle. The skin island of the saphenous flap is placed according to the distribution of the dominant perforators. If there are no dominant perforators, then the flap is designed over the distal sartorius, which is included in the flap. The length of the pedicle ranges from 5 to 15 cm and has a diameter of 1.5 to 2 mm.

The venous drainage includes the greater saphenous vein and the paired venae comitantes. The saphenous vein is used in microvascular transplantation.

The sensory nerve supply is from the anterior femoral cutaneous nerve, and the saphenous nerve innervates the upper portions and the lower portions of the flap, respectively.

The patient is positioned supine with the appropriate knee flexed and the hip rotated laterally. The sartorius is marked with a line from the anterior superior iliac spine to the medial condyle of the tibia. The skin paddle is centered over the distal aspect of the sartorius muscle. The incision is taken down to the anterior border of the sartorius, and the medial femoral cutaneous nerve is identified anterior to the muscle. The vein is found along the posterior aspect of the sartorius muscle. The artery is identified by incising the deep fascia and dissecting off the vastus medialis muscle. The dominant perforators are then assessed and used to determine cutaneous flap design. The sartorius muscle may either be divided or a portion of the muscle can be included to preserve the arterial supply to the skin paddle. The saphenous vein is divided. Proximally, 15 cm of pedicle length can be obtained, allowing for transposition. Donor sites less than 7 cm can be closed primarily with skin grafts needed for larger defects.

MUSCLE FLAPS

Sartorius Flap

The sartorius flap is a muscle or musculocutaneous flap that originates on the anterior superior iliac spine and inserts on the medial tibial condyle. The muscle is approximately $5 \times 40\ \text{cm}^2$ and functions as a lateral rotator and thigh flexor. The sartorius muscle has a type IV pattern of circulation and is supplied by six to seven branches of the superficial femoral artery. This muscle is expendable and may provide coverage to the groin, femoral vessels, and knee. It is most commonly used for muscle flap coverage of the femoral vessels during vascular surgery or groin dissection.

The venous supply is analogous to the arterial supply with several branches draining into the superficial femoral vein. The motor nerve to the sartorius muscle is the femoral nerve.

The distal sartorius can be divided from the insertion and transposed to cover a small medial knee defect. The donor site is easily closed primarily.

Vastus Lateralis

The vastus lateralis muscle originates on the intertrochanteric line, greater trochanter, gluteal tuberosity, and lateral intermuscular septum and inserts on the patella. The muscle is approximately $10 \times 26\ \text{cm}^2$ and can be palpated between the lateral margins of the rectus femoris and the biceps femoris.

The vastus lateralis muscle has a type I vascular pattern supply. The dominant pedicle is the descending branch of the lateral circumflex femoral artery. The dominant venous drainage is from the venae comitantes of the descending branch of the lateral circumflex femoral artery. The minor pedicles also have venae comitantes branches. There are also direct venous branches to the profunda femoris vein.

The motor supply is from the femoral nerve and is found at the proximal, medial muscle belly and is just inferior to the descending branch of the lateral circumflex femoral artery. The sensory nerve supplying the overlying skin is the lateral femoral cutaneous nerve.

Also, a distal flap can be designed based on the superior lateral genicular artery. This can be used to cover knee defects, however, it may be unreliable and use of the entire muscle may require microvascular anastomosis of the dominant pedicle to an acceptable distal donor vessel. The donor site may be closed primarily.

Vastus Medialis

The vastus medialis originates from the distal half of the intertrochanteric line, medial lip of the linea aspera, medial proximal supracondylar line, tendons of the adductor longus and adductor magnus muscles, and the medial intermuscular septum. The muscle inserts on the medial border of the patella and the quadriceps femoris mechanism and functions as a knee extensor. It is also expendable because of the function of the remaining quadriceps muscle. The muscle unit is approximately $15 \times 8\ cm^2$ and is located on the medial aspect of the thigh, medial to the rectus femoris and deep to the sartorius muscle. This muscle or musculocutaneous flap has useful applications for coverage of upper knee defects, based on its distal minor pedicle. The distal muscle can be transposed to close the superior aspect of the knee and can also be used to reconstruct the extensor mechanism of the knee. A V–Y myocutaneous advancement flap can be moved from the patella to the tibial tubercle. Another use for the vastus medialis muscle is for anterior and posterior middle thigh coverage.

The muscle has a type II pattern of circulation. The dominant pedicle is a branch of the superficial femoral artery. This vessel is 1–3 cm in length and enters the muscle medially between the middle and upper third of the muscle. There are other smaller branches directly off the superficial femoral artery. There is a 2-cm musculoarticular branch of the descending genicular artery that supplies the distal portion of the muscle. Based on this 2-cm minor pedicle, a branch from the superficial femoral artery, the distal portion of the vastus medialis can be divided to cover the knee.

The venous drainage is from the venae comitantes accompanying the arterial supply. The motor supply is from the femoral nerve and the sensation to the cutaneous portion of the flap is from the saphenous nerve. The motor branch accompanies the dominant vascular pedicle and enters the medial upper aspect of the muscle.

The patient is placed in the prone position. A line is drawn from the anterior superior iliac spine medial condyle of the femur, representing the sartorius. The vastus medialis muscle lies deep to the sartorius and medial to the rectus femoris. For muscle transposition, an incision is made in the anterolateral thigh. The distal muscle is elevated with preservation of the pedicle, located deep and medial to the muscle. The muscle is divided proximal to the most distal segmental branch and then can be transposed into an upper knee defect. A $20 \times 10\ cm^2$ skin island can be drawn between the rectus femoris and gracilis muscle on the midmedial thigh. A V–Y advancement flap can then be designed to be advanced distally over the medial upper thigh and knee after elevation of the muscle. The donor site is closed primarily.

MIDDLE THIRD RECONSTRUCTION

Soleus Flap

The most commonly used muscle for reconstruction of middle third defects is the soleus muscle flap. The lateral belly originates on the posterior surface of the body and head of the fibula, and the medial belly originates on the middle third of the tibia. The muscle inserts into the calcaneus after fusing with the gastrocnemius to form the Achilles tendon. The function of the muscle is plantar flexion of the foot. The soleus muscle is also responsible for the venous pump mechanism and functions in posture stabilization and slow gait. The muscle is expendable if at least one head of the gastrocnemius is preserved. The muscle is approximately 8×28 cm^2 and is located deep to the gastrocnemius in the superficial posterior compartment of the leg. Proximally the muscle heads are fused, but distally there is a septum dividing them. The muscle has applications for coverage of small- to moderate-size defects in the middle third of the lower extremity.

The soleus muscle has a type II pattern of circulation. The major segmental pedicles include the muscular branches of the popliteal artery, the proximal two branches of the posterior tibial artery, and the proximal two branches of the peroneal artery. There are also three or four minor pedicle branches from the posterior tibial artery. The major pedicles enter the muscle in the upper third of the muscle along the deep aspect. The posterior tibial artery branches enter medially and the peroneal branches enter laterally. The minor segmental branches are located along the distal medial border.

The venous drainage is from the venae comitantes accompanying the arterial supply. The motor nerve supply is from the posterior tibial and medial popliteal nerves.

The patient is placed in the supine position. The standard approach is through an incision 2 cm medial to the medial edge of the tibia taken down to the medial malleolus. The soleus muscle is found deep to the gastrocnemius muscle and plantaris tendon. The origin is partially divided off the tibia and the insertion is off the Achilles tendon. The posterior tibial artery is identified to avoid injury to the vessel. The distal segmental vessels are divided, and the muscle can be transposed into a middle third leg defect. Modifications to the soleus flap include a lateral approach and a hemisoleus flap. The donor site is closed primarily. Typically the lateral approach is not used because the fibula limits the arc of rotation. The posterior tibial artery is identified to avoid injury to the vessel. It is an expendable muscle with an acceptable donor site. The disadvantage to harvest of the soleus is that it is more difficult to dissect than the gastrocnemius, and the distal tip of the muscle may not survive. This muscle is also often involved in the zone of injury.

FASCIOCUTANEOUS FLAPS

Anterior Tibial Artery Flap

The anterior tibial artery flap is a fasciocutaneous flap located on the anterolateral aspect of the leg between the knee and lateral malleolus. Flaps with skin paddles of 6×18 cm^2 can be transposed proximally or distally. The standard flap is proximally based and will arc to provide coverage of the tibia. A reverse flap can be transposed to cover the lateral malleolus and proximal foot.

The dominant arterial pedicle is from septocutaneous branches of the anterior tibial artery. These 3–4 cm vessels are found lateral to the tibia and run between the tibialis anterior muscle and extensor digitorum longus in the proximal leg and the tibialis anterior and extensor hallucis longus in the distal leg. These vessels supply the skin of the anterolateral leg after transversing the deep fascia.

The venous drainage is from the venae comitantes accompanying the arterial supply. The sensory nerves are the common peroneal nerve to the superior portion and the superficial peroneal nerve to the inferior portion.

The patient is placed in the supine position, with a bump placed under the ipsilateral buttock to expose the lateral aspect of the lower leg. The flap is centered over a parallel line 2 cm anterior to the fibula between the head of the fibula and the lateral malleolus. The skin territory over the anterior compartment of the leg has a width of 3 to 8 cm and a length of 6 to 20 cm. A standard U-shaped flap can be designed along the upper third or middle third of the lower leg. After the vertical incisions are completed the fasciocutaneous perforators are identified deep to the fascia at the level of the intermuscular septum. The tibialis anterior and extensor digitorum longus are anterior, and the soleus and peroneus brevis muscles are posterior. The septocutaneous perforators are preserved at the flap base. The peritenon over the peroneus longus tendon and the periosteum over the fibula are preserved with distal flap elevation. The distal anterior intermuscular septum is divided to allow for flap rotation 90° to the anterior tibia. A reverse flap can be rotated 180° to reach the ankle or foot. In addition, the fascia without skin may be utilized for tissue coverage. Incorporating the superficial peroneal nerve can create a sensate flap. The donor site may be closed primarily if the width of the flap is under 4 cm, otherwise a skin graft may be required.

Peroneal Artery Flap

The peroneal artery flap is a fasciocutaneous flap located on the lateral leg over the fibula. The maximal area of tissue that can be transferred is approximately 20×8 cm^2 and includes the tissue between the lateral aspect of the gastrocnemius and tibialis anterior muscle and between the head of the fibula and the lateral malleolus. The standard design for middle third of the leg coverage is a U-shaped flap with the apex at the posterior lateral ankle. A distally based flap with the apex at the level of the proximal fibula can also arc to the middle third of the leg. The flap can also be used for microvascular transplantation.

The dominant pedicle consists of five to six segmental septocutaneous arteries arising from the peroneal artery. These 3-cm branches pass through the posterior peroneal septum between the styloid process and the lateral malleolus of the fibula, approximately 9–20 cm inferior to the styloid process. Minor pedicles include musculocutaneous perforators from the peroneal artery, sural artery, and anterior tibial arteries.

The venous drainage is from the venae comitantes accompanying the arterial supply. The sensory nerve supply is from the superficial peroneal nerve, which supplies sensation to the lateral leg. This nerve is located deep to the fascia between the extensor digitorum longus and peroneal muscles.

The patient is placed in the lateral decubitus position. The skin paddle is designed over the center of the posterior edge of the fibula and an incision is taken down through the deep fascia. The tibialis anterior, extensor digitorum, and peroneus tertius muscles are identified in the anterior compartment. The gastrocnemius and soleus muscles are identified in the posterior compartment. The anterior intermuscular septum is divided between the extensor digitorum longus and peroneus tertius muscles. The dominant segmental pedicles are identified along the anterior surface of the posterior intermuscular septum, located in the groove between the peroneus brevis and the flexor hallucis longus muscle. Flap elevation is begun at the inferior flap edge up to the flap base with preservation of the pedicle. The flap may then be rotated 90° into a middle leg defect. Skin grafts are used to cover the donor site.

Posterior Tibial Artery Flap

The posterior tibial artery flap is a fasciocutaneous flap located on the medial aspect of the lower leg from the knee to the medial malleolus. The maximal area of tissue that can be transferred is approximately $6 \times 18\ cm^2$. The standard flap is a U-shaped flap, which is elevated from the lower or middle third of the medial leg and with a superiorly based pedicle. A U-shaped flap based on the distal blood supply can also be designed for coverage of the lower or middle third of the leg.

The major blood supply is six to seven septocutaneous perforators of the posterior tibial artery, located just behind the posterior border of the tibia. These 2–4 cm run between the soleus and the flexor digitorum longus and usually are larger more proximally. There is a network between perforators so the flap can be based on one perforator.

The venous drainage is from the venae comitantes accompanying the arterial supply. The sensory nerve supply is from the saphenous nerve. The patient is placed in the supine position with the leg externally rotated. A U-shaped flap is drawn centered over a vertical line located over the anterior medial leg between the medial edge of the tibia and the anterior edge of the Achilles tendon distally and the gastrocnemius muscle proximally. A flap base/length ratio of 3:1 is considered safe. An incision is made along the anterior or posterior edge and the septocutaneous vessels are identified at the base of the flap deep to the fascia. Elevation of the flap requires division of the distal perforating vessels between the soleus and flexor digitorum longus muscles. The superiorly based flap can then be transposed into a middle or lower third leg defect. A distally based flap with the apex below the knee can also be rotated into a middle leg defect. The donor site will require a skin graft.

Sural Artery Flap

The sural artery flap is a fasciocutaneous flap located between the popliteal fossa and the midline raphe between the medial and lateral heads of the gastrocnemius muscle. The maximal area of tissue that can be transferred is approximately

$20 \times 12\ cm^2$. The standard flap is a U-shaped flap with the apex in the midposterior leg centered over the midline raphe between the heads of the gastrocnemius. After elevation, the flap will reach defects in the knee, popliteal fossa, and the upper third of the leg. The flap can also be designed as an island flap, reversed flap, or for use in microvascular transplantation.

The dominant pedicle is a direct cutaneous artery arising from the popliteal artery. This sural artery branch is approximately 3 cm long and is found between the heads of the gastrocnemius and then located inferior and superficial to the gastrocnemius muscle. The minor pedicle is a musculocutaneous perforating artery from the gastrocnemius muscle. The venous drainage is from the lesser saphenous vein. The sensory nerve is the medial sural cutaneous nerve. This is a branch of the tibial nerve and accompanies the lesser saphenous vein and artery.

The patient is placed in a prone or lateral decubitus position. A line is drawn from the posterior midline in the popliteal fossa to the midportion of the heel. A U-shaped skin flap is designed with the apex placed inferiorly. A Doppler probe is used to locate the pedicles' course. An incision is taken down through the fascia. The distal saphenous vein and sural nerve are divided. The flap is then elevated proximally in the subfascial plane between the deep fascia and the gastrocnemius muscle. The pedicle and lesser saphenous vein are then identified in the proximal aspect of the flap. The flap can then be transposed to the knee, popliteal fossa, and upper third of the leg. The flap can also be designed as an island or reverse flap. A skin graft is usually required for coverage of the donor site.

MUSCLE FLAPS

Extensor Digitorum Longus Flap

The extensor digitorum longus muscle originates on the lateral tibial condyle of the anterior surface of the fibula and the interosseous membrane. The muscle inserts on the middle and distal phalanges of the four lateral toes and its function is to extend the four lateral toes. The extensor digitorum longus muscle is $4 \times 35\ cm^2$ and is located on the anterolateral aspect of the leg, lateral to the tibialis anterior. This muscle is expendable because the extensor digitorum brevis muscle will provide proximal interphalangeal joint extension. Because distal interphalangeal extension will be lost, the functional muscle-tendon unit may be preserved with elevation of the flap, resulting in a transferable $5 \times 8\ cm^2$ muscle. This muscle flap has applications in coverage of defects of the middle and lower thirds of the tibia.

The muscle has a type IV pattern of circulation. There are 8 to 10 segmental arterial branches arising from the anterior tibial artery. These 1- to 2-cm branches are located on the medial aspect of the muscle and can be found between the extensor digitorum longus and the tibialis anterior muscles. The segmental blood supply limits the arc of rotation. The skin overlying the muscle can be utilized in an anterior tibial artery flap.

The venous drainage is from the venae comitantes accompanying the arterial supply. The motor nerve supply is from the deep peroneal nerve. The patient is placed in a supine position. A line is drawn from 2 cm lateral to the lateral border of the tibia below the knee distal to a point 5 cm superior to the lateral malleolus. An incision is then made along this line and taken down through the fascia. The tibialis anterior is retracted medially to identify the extensor digitorum longus and the vascular pedicles. A superiorly based flap will provide coverage of the lower third of the anterior tibia after the lower three or four vascular pedicles are ligated and the distal muscle is divided. An inferiorly based flap will provide coverage of the middle third of the tibia after the proximal three or four vascular pedicles are ligated and the muscle is divided superiorly. The majority of the muscle can be mobilized without ligating the segmental pedicles and then advanced onto the tibia. Skin grafts are placed onto the exposed muscle and the donor site closed directly.

Extensor Hallucis Longus Flap

The extensor hallucis longus muscle originates on the anterior aspect of the midfibula and the interosseous septum and inserts on the distal phalanx of the great toe. It extends the great toe but is expendable because of the function of the extensor digitorum brevis. Usually the flap is elevated preserving the functional tendon unit. The muscle is approximately 3×24 cm^2 and lies deep to the tibialis anterior and the extensor digitorum longus muscle. This pure muscle flap is small and is usually used in conjunction with a tibialis anterior flap or extensor digitorum flap. A superiorly based flap will cover lower third defects. An inferiorly based flap will cover small distal tibia defects.

The muscle has a type IV pattern of circulation. The major segmental pedicles are six to eight arterial branches from the anterior tibial artery. These 1- to 2-cm branches enter the muscle along the medial aspect of the muscle. Due to the segmental nature of the blood supply the arc of rotation is limited.

The venous drainage is from the venae comitantes accompanying the arterial supply. The motor nerve supply is from the deep peroneal nerve.

The patient is placed in the supine position. A line is drawn from the tibial tubercle down to a point 4 cm superior to the lateral malleolus. This line is incised and the tibial anterior and the extensor digitorum longus are exposed. The extensor hallucis longus muscle is identified as the extensor digitorum longus muscle is retracted laterally. Retracting the muscle laterally identifies the pedicle and nerve supply. The distal musculotendinous fibers are divided above the extensor retinaculum and two to three distal segmental pedicles are ligated. A portion of muscle is elevated from the interosseous membrane, allowing for transposition of the muscle into a small middle third defect. An inferiorly based flap based on the distal two to three segmental pedicles allows for transposition into small middle third leg defects. The donor site is closed primarily.

Flexor Digitorum Longus Flap

The flexor digitorum longus muscle originates on the posterior surface of the tibia and inserts on the base of the distal phalanges of the second, third, fourth, and fifth toes. It functions to flex the distal phalanges and is expendable if the muscle insertion is not divided and the flexor digitorum brevis muscle is left intact. The muscle is approximately $5 \times 40\ cm^2$ and is located medial to the tibia and between the soleus and tibialis posterior muscles. This small pure muscle flap has limited applications for coverage of the middle and lower third of the leg.

The muscle has a type IV pattern of circulation. The major segmental pedicles are 10 to 12 arterial branches from the posterior tibial artery. These 1- to 2-cm vessels enter the muscle along the posterior aspect of the deep muscle surface. Due to the segmental nature of the blood supply the arc of rotation is limited.

The venous drainage is from the venae comitantes accompanying the arterial supply. The motor nerve supply is from the muscular branch of the tibial nerve.

The patient is placed in the supine position. A line is drawn from the medial border of the tibia to the posterior medial malleolus, along the medial border of the tibia. An incision is made and the flexor digitorum longus muscle is identified deep to the soleus muscle. The tendon is divided distally posterior to the medial malleolus and between the tendons of the tibialis posterior and the flexor hallucis longus. One or two distal segmental perforators are divided and the muscle can be transposed posteriorly to the middle third of the leg or anteriorly to the lower third of the leg. An inferiorly based flap based on the distal perforators can be transposed for coverage of middle third small defects after the muscle origin is divided along with three or four proximal segmental vessels. Because the muscle is small and has a segmental blood supply it is usually used along with a soleus muscle flap. The donor site may be closed primarily.

Peroneus Longus Flap

The peroneus longus muscle originates on the upper lateral fibula and inserts on the lateral base of the first metatarsal and medial cuneiform bones. It functions to evert and plantarflex the foot. The muscle is expendable if the peroneus brevis and tertius muscles are left intact. The muscle is approximately $4 \times 10\ cm^2$ and is located in the lateral leg compartment between the fibula and posterior foot. It is posterior to the fibula, anterior to the extensor digitorum longus, and superficial to the peroneus brevis muscle. The functional muscle-tendon unit may be preserved with elevation of the flap. This small muscle flap has applications for coverage of the middle and proximal thirds of the tibial defects.

The muscle has a type II pattern of circulation. The major segmental pedicle is a muscular branch of the peroneal artery. This 3-cm vessel is located on the proximal deep surface of the muscle, arising from beneath the flexor hallucis longus muscle. The minor pedicles are muscular branches of the anterior tibial artery. These smaller branches supply the distal two-thirds of the muscle.

The venous drainage is from the venae comitantes accompanying the arterial supply. The motor supply to the muscle is the motor branch of the superficial peroneal nerve. This branch of the common peroneal nerve enters the muscle on its deep surface near the muscle origin. The superficial peroneal nerve also supplies the skin of the lateral muscle compartment.

The patient is placed in the lateral decubitus position. A line is drawn on the lateral leg 2 cm below the fibula head down to the posterior aspect of the lateral malleolus. The incision is taken down to the level of the muscle, and the peroneus longus is identified between the extensor digitorum longus muscle anteriorly and the soleus muscle laterally. The tendon insertion is divided and the muscle elevated proximally with preservation of the major pedicle. A narrow skin island may be incorporated with the flap over the muscle. The muscle will arc 90° to the middle third of the anterior leg. The donor site is closed primarily.

Tibialis Anterior Flap

The tibialis anterior muscle originates on the lateral condyle and upper lateral surface of the tibia and interosseous membrane. It inserts on the medial cuneiform and base of the first metatarsal. It functions to dorsiflex and invert the foot and it is not expendable. The muscle is approximately $4 \times 25\ cm^2$ and is located lateral to the tibia. The functional muscle-tendon unit may be preserved with elevation of the flap. This muscle flap has applications for coverage of the middle and upper third of the lower leg.

The muscle has a type IV pattern of circulation. The major segmental pedicles are 8 to 12 arterial muscular branches arising from the anterior tibial artery. The anterior tibial artery is found between the tibialis anterior and the extensor digitorum longus muscles. These 1- to 2-cm vessels enter the muscle from the lateral deep aspect of the muscle. Due to the segmental blood supply of the muscle, the arc of rotation is limited.

The venous drainage is from the venae comitantes accompanying the arterial supply. The motor nerve is from the deep peroneal nerve. The patient is placed in the supine position. A line is drawn 1 cm from the lateral border of the tibia from the knee down to the ankle. An incision is taken down to the level of the muscle. The segmental vessels are identified and a portion of muscle is split in the longitudinal plane allowing for preservation of function. A 1- to 1.5-cm thick muscle flap can then be mobilized to cover an exposed proximal tibia. A portion of muscle and distal segmental vessels can be divided distally and transposed 90° for small defects of the middle and upper third of the lower leg. The donor site is closed primarily.

FREE TISSUE TRANSFER

The role of free tissue transfer for reconstruction of proximal and middle third defects is useful particularly in wounds associated with severe trauma. Lower extremity injuries with significant bone or tissue loss may require free flap coverage. The lack of local reconstructive options, i.e., gastrocnemius and soleus, or loss of the primary flap usually requires coverage from a distant source. Free tissue transfer for soft-tissue reconstruction of the lower extremity is beyond the scope of this chapter and will be dealt with in another section and is mentioned for completeness.

TISSUE EXPANSION

Tissue expansion is another option for soft-tissue reconstruction of the lower extremity. The use of tissue expansion is usually in the setting of delayed reconstruction (i.e., scar removal). The soft tissue surrounding the defect can be expanded by placement of tissue expanders. Use of tissue expansion depends on the quality of skin, the size of the defect, and the location. When evaluating a patient for tissue expansion, the geometry of the wound is critical along with the geometry of the expander. As the soft tissue is expanded, a capsule forms, and this capsule contributes to the blood supply and therefore should be left intact during the secondary procedure, removal of the expander and soft-tissue reconstruction. Advancement of skin is mostly in a transverse fashion around the leg and not axial along the length of the leg. Tissue expansion allows tissue of like color and texture, sensation, and hair-bearing quality with decreased donor site scar. Patients undergo slow expansion, often taking two to three months. Tissue expanders can have either an internal or an external valve, and sometimes patients can be taught to do expansion at home.

Tissue expansion is associated with many complications, including extrusion, pain, hematoma, seroma, deflation, valve problems, leakage, and neuropraxia. There is an increased risk of infection with tissue expansion and extrusion, particularly in the lower extremity. In addition, the area to be expanded may be significantly fibrosed from the prior injury and may not tolerate the expansion process. Finally, the placement of a tissue expander surrounding an open wound is contraindicated. Taken together, the role for tissue expansion in the management of lower extremity wounds is limited.

WOUND VACUUM-ASSISTED CLOSURE

Another option for soft tissue closure is the wound vacuum-assisted closure (VAC). The wound VAC device applies a negative pressure to the wound. Argenta has shown an increased rate in granulation formation with egress of large volumes of edematous fluid for massive soft-tissue wounds. It has shown some success in treatment of overimplanted orthopedic hardware and dehisced wounds. Therefore, the wound VAC can be used as an adjunct for management of lower extremity soft-tissue trauma. We have had some favorable results in our institution with use of the VAC for complex lower extremity reconstruction following failed free tissue transfer and as an aid to complex wound closure.

COMPLICATIONS IN RECONSTRUCTION

Lower extremity reconstruction can be a challenge to even the most experienced plastic surgeon and can be fraught with complications. Neat showed a 34% incidence of major complications with soft-tissue reconstruction. Lower extremity reconstruction can be problematic because it is often difficult to determine the "zone of injury" in the area to be reconstructed. This can result in flap loss or failure. Another reason is for flap loss is technical error, such as poor flap design. Infections can result in flap failure, particularly if the patient has or develops chronic osteomyelitis. Even patients who have adequate soft-tissue coverage can go on to develop chronic osteomyelitis and eventually need amputation. Infection and necrosis often occur as a result of inadequate debridement of the bone and soft tissue. Salvage of flaps is sometimes successful with readvancement of the flaps; however, often additional reconstruction may be done with a secondary flap or free tissue transfer.

CONCLUSION

The incidence of lower extremity wounds reconstruction is increasing, and all efforts should be directed towards functional limb salvage. It is important to maintain a team approach with orthopedic surgeons, vascular surgeons, and plastic surgeons working together to treat these complex wounds. As described above there are many options available to the plastic surgeon for lower extremity reconstruction. The gastrocnemius and soleus muscles continue to be workhorses for upper third defects and middle third defects, respectively. When local or regional flaps fail, it is often necessary to employ free tissue transfer for reconstruction.

REFERENCES

1. Aldea PA, Shaw WW. Lower extremity nerve injuries. Clin Plast Surg 1986; 13:691.
2. Armante J, Costa H, Ruies J, Soares R. A new distally based fasciocutaneous flap of the leg. Br J Plast Surg 1986; 39(A):33.
3. Arnold PG, Mixter RC. Making the most of the gastrocnemius muscle. Plast End Reconstr Surg 1983; 72:38.
4. Arnold PG, Prunes-Carillo F. Vastus medialis muscle flap for functional closure of the exposed knee joint. Plast Reconstr Surg 1981; 68:69.
5. Borges Filho PT, Neves RI, Manders EK, et al. Soft tissue expansion in lower extremity reconstruction. Clin Plast Surg 1991; 18:593.
6. Byrd HS, Spicer TE, Cierny G III. Management of open tibial fractures. Plast Reconstr Surg 1985; 76:719.
7. Chang N, Mathes SJ, Calderon W. Comparison of the effect of bacterial inoculation musculocutaneous and fasciocutaneous flaps. Plast Reconstr Surg 1986; 7:785–793.
8. Cierny G III, Byrd HS, Jones RE. Primary vs. delayed soft tissue coverage for severe open tibia fractures: a comparison of results. Clin Orthoped 1983; 54:178.

9. Ciemy G III, Wornom I III, Nahai F. Reconstruction of difficult wounds of the lower extremity. Prob Gen Surg 1989; 6:699.
10. De La Playa R, Arroyo JM, Vasconez LO. Upper transverse rectus abdominus flap: the flag flap. Ann Plast Surg 1984; 12:410.
11. Dowden RV, McCraw JB. The vastus lateralis muscle flap: technique and applications. Ann Plast Surg 1980; 4:396.
12. Elshay NI. Cover of the exposed knee joint by the lateral head of the gastrocnemius. Br J Plast Surg 1978; 31:136.
13. Fix JR, Vasconez LO. Fasciocutaneous flaps m reconstruction of the lower extremity. Clin Plast Surg 1991; 18:571.
14. Filho PB, Neves RI, Manders EK, et al. Soft tissue expansion m lower extremity reconstruction. Clin Plast Surg 1991; 18:593.
15. Francel TJ, Vander Kolk CA, Hoopes JE, et al. Microvascular soft-tissue transplantation for reconstruction of acute open tibial fractures: timing of coverage and long-term functional results. Plast Reconstr Surg 1992; 89:478–487.
16. Given KS, Drew GS. Basic principles involving the management of tissue loss in the lower extremity, including muscle and musculocutaneous flaps. In: Georgiade GS, et al., eds. Textbook of Plastic, Maxillofacial and Reconstructive Surgery. 2nd ed. Baltimore: Williams and Wilkins, 1992:1299–1305.
17. Godina M. Early microsurgical reconstruction of complex trauma of extremities. Clin Plast Surg 1986; 13:619.
18. Gu Y, Wu M, Li H. Lateral lower leg skin flap. Ann Plast Surg 1985; 15:319.
19. Gustilo RB, Mendoza RM, Williams DN. Problems in the management of type III open fractures: a new classification system. J Trauma 1988; 24:742.
20. Guzman-Stein G, Fix JR, Vasconez LO. Muscle flap coverage for the lower extremity. Clin Plast Surg 1991; 18:545.
21. Guy M. Extremities. In: Nordstrom RA, ed. Tissue Expansion. Boston: Butterworth Heinnemann, 1996:131–135.
22. Hallock GG. Reconstruction for lower extremity trauma. In: Goldwyn RM, Cohen MN, eds. The Unfavorable Result in Plastic Surgery. 3rd ed. Philadelphia: Lippincott Williams and Wilkins, 2001:833–841.
23. Hallock GG. Relative donor site morbidity of muscle and fascial flaps. Plast Reconstr Surg 1993; 92:70–76.
24. Heller L, Levin LS. Lower extremity microsurgical reconstruction. Plast Reconstr Surg 2001; 108:1029.
25. Kasabian AK, King NS. Lower extremity reconstruction. In: Aston, Beasley, Theme, eds. Grabb and Smiths Plastic Surgery. Philadelphia: Lippincott Raven, 1991:1031–1047.
26. Kennedy JP. Soft tissue injury. In: Kennedy JP, Blaisdell FW, eds. Extremity Trauma. New York: Thieme, 1992:16–28.
27. Koshima I, Endou T, Soeda S, Yamasaki M. The free or pedicled saphenous flap. Ann Plast Surg 1988; 21:369.
28. Li Z, Liu K, Lin Y, Li L. Lateral sural cutaneous artery island flap in the treatment of soft tissue defects of the knee. Br J Plastic Surg 1990; 43:546.
29. Long CD, Granick MS, Solomon MP. The cross-leg flap revisited. Ann Plast Surg 1993; 30:560.
30. Mahoney J. Salvage of the infected groin vascular graft with muscle flaps. Ann Plast Surg 1989; 22:252.

31. Mandel MA. Management of lower extremity degloving injuries. Ann Plast Surg 1981; 6:1.
32. Mathes SJ, Alpert BS, Chang N. Use of the muscle flap in chronic osteomyelitis experimental and clinical correlation. Plast Reconstr Surg 1982; 69:815.
33. Mathes SJ, McCraw JB, Vasconez LO. Muscle transposition flaps for coverage of lower extremity defects: anatomical considerations. Surg Clin North Am 1974; 54:1337.
34. Mathes SJ, Nahai F. Clinical Atlas of Muscle and Musculocutaneous Flaps. St. Louis: CV Mosby, 1979.
35. Mathes SJ, Nahai F. Reconstructive Surgery: Principles, Anatomy & Technique. New York: Churchill Livingstone, 1997.
36. Mathes SJ, Vasconez LO, Jurkiewicz MJ. Extension and further application of muscle flap transposition. Plast Reconstr Surg 1977; 60:6.
37. McCraw JB, Arnold PG. McCraw and Arnold's Atlas of Muscle and Musculocutaneous Flaps. Norfolk: Hampton Press, 1986.
38. Neale HW, Stem PC, N Kreflein JJ, et al. Complications of muscle flap transposition for traumatic defects of the leg. Plast Reconstr Surg 1983:72:512.
39. Ponten B. The fasciocutaneous flap: its use in soft tissue defects of the lower leg. Br J Plast Surg 1981; 34:215.
40. Rocha JF, Gilbert A, Masquelet A, Yusif NJ, Sanger JR, Matloub HS. The anterior tibial artery flap: anatomic study and clinical applications. Plast Reconstr Surg 1987; 79:396.
41. Serafin D, Voci V. Reconstruction of the lower extremity microsurgical composite tissue transplantation. Clin Plast Surg 1983; 10:55.
42. Yaremchuk MF. Acute management of severe soft tissue damage accompanying open fractures of the lower extremity. Clin Plast Surg 1986; 13:621.
43. Yaremchuk MF. Concepts in soft tissue management. In: Yaremchuk ND, Burgess AR, Brumback RJ, eds. Lower Extremity Salvage and Reconstruction. New York: Elsevier Science 1939:95–104.

7

Microsurgical Repair of Complex Soft-Tissue Defects

Jonathan Fisher
Division of Plastic Surgery, Miller School of Medicine, University of Miami, Miami, Florida, U.S.A.

Rajeev Venugopal
Department of Surgery, University of the West Indies, Jamaica, West Indies

Milton B. Armstrong
Division of Plastic Surgery, Miller School of Medicine, University of Miami, Miami, Florida, U.S.A.

Lower extremity reconstruction presents the plastic surgeon with complex problems of not only form, but also of function. Regardless of the etiology of the lower extremity defect—be it secondary to trauma, infection, vascular insufficiency, or tumor—the extent of the tissue deficit often dictates a shift in traditional thinking about progression along a reconstructive ladder. When conceptualizing a reconstruction, use of the reconstructive ladder, with a stepwise advancement from more simple to increasingly complex reconstructive options, forces the plastic surgeon to evaluate and justify the added complexity and theoretical added risks at each successive rung on the ladder. In lower extremity reconstruction, issues of limb salvage, expediency of rehabilitation, extensiveness of defect, and location of defect form clear indications for moving directly to the highest rung of the ladder: microvascular free-tissue transfer.

HISTORY OF MICROVASCULAR SURGERY

Plastic surgical flap techniques have existed for at least 5000 years. The Indian text Sushrata Samhita (ca. 3000 B.C.) contains a description of nasal reconstruction using locoregional flaps (1). Further advances in knowledge of anatomy, physiology, and the applied sciences led to the development of modern medicine. Progression of the pure sciences and the introduction of the scientific method allowed the evolution of surgical tools and the methodology required to utilize them effectively.

It was the invention and application of microscopy to surgery that inevitably led to the furtherance of microvascular surgical practice over the past 45 years. The ancient Egyptians are reported to have understood the principles of magnification (2). The first microscope was invented by Zacharias and Hans Janseen in 1590 (3). Advances in lens quality and optics led, eventually, to the construction of the first purpose-built medical scope by Carl Zeiss.

Nylen, an otolaryngologist, performed the first surgical procedure using a monocular microscope in 1920. Further improvements over the next 40 years, including binocular microscopy, beam-splitting to make surgical assistance possible, and cooler fiberoptics, as well as the development of specialized instruments by Castro-Viejo and others, facilitated the birth of modern microvascular surgery (2).

In 1960, Jacobson and Suarez used the operating microscope for the anastomosis of blood vessels (4). The use of the microscope allowed reliable anastomosis and a 100% patency rate in blood vessels ranging from 1.6 to 3.2 mm. Over the next four decades, increased knowledge of flap anatomy and increasing experience in the field of microsurgery led to a rapid expansion in the microvascular armamentarium (Table 1).

Table 1 Landmark Cases in Microvascular Surgery

Common cutaneous flaps		
Kaplan et al.	1973	Groin flap to intraoral site
Daniel and Taylor	1973	Hypogastric flap to lower extremity
O'Brien and Shaunmugan	1973	Dorsalis pedis flap
Guffan et al.	1978	Radial forearm flap
Ackland	1979	Extended groin flap
Katsoros	1982	Lateral arm flap
Gilbert and Teot	1982	Scapular flap
Harii	1983	Scalp flap
Muscle free flaps		
Tamai et al.	1950	Free rectus flap in dogs
Baudet et al.	1976	Axillary/latissimus dorsi flap
Harii et al.	1976	Gracilis flap
Hill et al.	1978	Tensor fascia lata flap
Manktelow et al.	1978	Functional gracilis transplant
Osseous free flaps		
McKee	1970	Rib for mandibular defect

(*Continued*)

Table 1 Landmark Cases in Microvascular Surgery (*Continued*)

Taylor et al.	1975	Vascularized fibula
Taylor et al.	1976	Vascularized iliac bone
Visceral transplants		
Seidenberg	1959	Canine jejunal transplant
Hiebert and Cummings	1961	Gastric antrum for esophageal reconstruction
Nakayama et al.	1964	Stapled transfer
Peters et al.	1971	Jejeunal transplant
McLean and Bunke	1972	Omentum to scalp defect
Replantation		
Kleinert and Kasdan	1963	Digit revascularization
Chen, Chien, and Pao	1963	Replantation at forearm
Malt and McKhann	1964	Replantations at arm level
Komatsu and Tamai	1965	Replantation of amputated digit
Cobbett	1969	First toe-to-hand transfer
Cohen	1974	Microvascular penile replantation
Miller et al.	1976	Replantation of scalp avulsion with vein grafts
Norman et al.	1976	Reattachment of upper lip and nose
Mathes et al.	1984	Vascularized transplant of metatarsal joint to metacarpal joint
Pennington et al.	1988	Reattachment of avulsed ear with vein grafts
Dubernard et al.	1998	First hand allotransplant

Source: From Ref. 2.

Advances in microsurgical technique have not only increased the success rates from around 70% in the 1960s to greater than 90% (5), but also have allowed reconstructive surgeons to shift their focus and their endpoints from mere salvage of tissue toward more functional and esthetic outcomes.

GENERAL CONSIDERATIONS

Prior to performing a free-tissue transfer repair, the surgeon must first evaluate the patient's overall candidacy for surgery. Use of free-tissue transfer has been described in both a pediatric setting and in the elderly (6). Ozkan et al. (7) describe a 25% medical complication rate and a 5.4% overall surgical mortality rate in free-flap patients over 50. The patient's preoperative medical condition was found to be the most significant prognostic factor. The authors feel that free-tissue transfer is an acceptable option for the elderly, and recommend careful patient selection and anticipation of postsurgical problems in higher-risk patients.

When deciding which type of free flap one will use for lower extremity reconstruction, one must contemplate several factors: the size and type of tissue defect, the size of the zone of injury, the necessary pedicle length, donor-site morbidity, and the esthetics of the reconstruction. The first decision to be made is whether the free flap will consist solely of one tissue type—a pure muscle, skin, fascia, or bone flap—or whether it will be a composite flap made up of two or more tissue types.

The size, shape, and volume of the defect will be primary determinants of flap choice. For defects that require primarily skin coverage or skin resurfacing, voluminous myocutaneous flaps like a free rectus flap are not as appropriate as smaller pure cutaneous or fasciocutaneous flaps. If there is a large cutaneous deficiency, flaps like the free rectus flap and the latissimus dorsi flap, which offer larger skin paddles, prove useful and can be used to fill volume defects with their bulky muscular components. If filling a dead space is the primary goal, muscle flaps can be harvested alone without an overlying skin paddle. An additional benefit of muscle flaps is that they provide additional vascularity to the wound. Finally, free osseous flaps can be used to provide bony reconstruction in cases where there is a skeletal defect.

The zone of injury includes the overall area of direct tissue damage but often extends well beyond the limits of the visualized wound. The mechanism of injury is the key factor in determining the magnitude of collateral tissue damage. Crush injuries and high-energy wounds (i.e., high-velocity gunshot wounds) often have extensive zones of injury which may take several days to completely demarcate. It is postulated that the inflammatory response to injury increases vessel friability and perivascular scar tissue, which can contribute to a higher failure rate of free-tissue transfer (8). The majority of authors advocate proximal dissection of the recipient vessels and anastomosis of the donor vessels well outside of the zone of injury. Park et al. argue that vessels distal to the zone of injury can be used as recipients, or even for reverse flow, if they are proven to have ample perfusion (9).

Required pedicle length is an important factor in flap choice. The necessary pedicle length is in turn determined by the location of the defect and the size of the zone of injury. In favorable cases, where the defect is small, and there are good close recipient vessels, pedicle length is not important. In other cases, where there may be extensive soft-tissue loss or vascular trauma, a flap with a longer pedicle is preferred (latissimus dorsi, rectus, or serratus flaps). In severe cases, vein grafts can be used to augment pedicle length, with less predictable results (10).

Donor-site morbidity should not be overlooked when considering free-tissue transfer. The surgeon must weigh the benefits of obtaining vascularized tissue against the relatively high complication rate. In lower extremity reconstruction, often the need for good tissue is so compelling that donor-site morbidity takes a less important role in the decision-making process. Complications such as unsightly scar, seroma, hematoma, or an abdominal bulge may be inconvenient for the patient, but are minor issues when considering limb salvage or major reconstruction. It is, however, important to educate patients about potential donor-site morbidity, provide them with a good rationale for the harvesting of distant tissue, and involve them in the decision-making process.

Finally, the esthetics of the reconstruction should be considered. As microsurgical technique has progressed, as success rates have improved, and as the options for reconstruction have increased in number, esthetic concerns have shifted from being only a secondary consideration to being part of the process of choosing the ideal flap for reconstruction. The size, shape, and bulk of the flap should be tailored to match the recipient defect when possible. Heller and Levin (8) even suggest that free-tissue transfer can be used for esthetic resurfacing of lower extremities and that this constitutes the "highest rung" on the reconstructive ladder.

RECONSTRUCTIVE OPTIONS BY LOCATION

The use of free-tissue transfer is clearly indicated in salvageable limbs with massive soft tissue or bony loss. The mechanism of injury, size of defect, and constituent parts of the defect are factors that may obviate the use of local or regional flaps for coverage. The availability of locoregional options also varies by location in the lower extremity, and it is often the location of the defect which is the primary determinant of type of reconstruction chosen.

Thigh

Defects involving the thigh usually do not require free-tissue transfer for reconstruction. Unless there is massive tissue loss, there is usually adequate soft tissue which can be advanced or rotated into the defect. Groin defects or exposure of the femoral vessels can usually be addressed with local flaps (sartorius flap) or pedicled locoregional flaps (VRAM).

Proximal Third

There are abundant local muscle flap options for coverage in the proximal third. The workhorses of the proximal third are the medial and lateral gastocnemius flaps and the proximally based soleus flap. These flaps—and other options—will be discussed elsewhere in this text. Free-tissue transfer can be used if the zone of injury is extensive enough to preclude local coverage.

Middle Third

Numerous muscle flaps and fasciocutaneous flaps can be designed for coverage of defects in the middle third of the leg. The proximally based soleus flap offers the most extensive coverage, but other local flaps can be used for smaller defects. Free-tissue transfer is often appropriate for middle third injuries with associated high-energy open tibial fractures when local muscle does not appear reliable or when soft-tissue defects exceed the coverage capacity of locoregional flaps.

Distal Third

Reconstruction of distal third primarily is accomplished with the use of free-tissue transfer. The availability of locoregional tissue for coverage is limited and the majority of options are only capable of covering relatively small defects. Fasciocutaneous flaps, like the reverse sural artery flap, can be useful for distal coverage, but may not be available in cases with extensive tissue loss.

Foot

Reconstruction of the foot represents a more difficult problem. Weight-bearing surfaces are prone to breakdown and should be reconstructed with thick plantar tissue if at all possible. Local advancement and pedicle flaps are preferable to free-tissue transfer. Free-tissue transfer can be used for large defects, in salvage cases, and in cases where some padding over bone is required. Weight bearing can be successfully achieved in the majority of patients (5).

TRAUMA

The first decision that must be made in massive lower extremity trauma is whether the limb should be salvaged or whether the patient should undergo a primary amputation. The primary goal of limb salvage is to give the patient a functional extremity with good rehabilitation potential. If reconstruction cannot provide a functional extremity, then it is better to perform an amputation, as return to function may be achieved sooner (8).

The extent of soft-tissue damage and the neurovascular status are the most important criteria for determining whether or not to perform a primary amputation. Mangled limbs with extensive soft-tissue injury and loss may not be candidates for functional salvage. Vascular injury with ischemia time greater than six hours has been shown to lead to poor outcomes. Nerve damage leading to a nonfunctional or insensate foot may also preclude reconstruction and has been posited to be an absolute indication for limb amputation (11).

Classification of Open Tibial Fractures

Efforts have been made to classify open tibial fractures based on their severity. There is a wide spectrum of injury in open tibial fractures and while the Gustilo and Byrd classifications are descriptive, these classification schemes serve mostly as guidelines to aid in surgical thinking (12,13).

The Gustilo classification (12) separates open tibial fractures into three main types. Type I injuries have little soft-tissue damage and have a wound less than 1 cm in diameter. Type II injuries have a wound larger than 1 cm, but still do not have extensive soft-tissue injury. In the majority of cases, type I and II injuries can be treated with locoregional flaps.

Type III injuries have more extensive soft-tissue damage and are separated into three subtypes based on the extent of that damage. Type IIIA injuries have adequate soft-tissue coverage. Type IIIB injuries have periosteal stripping and bone exposure. Type IIIC injuries have vascular compromise and require arterial repair. Depending upon the extent of the bony and soft-tissue damage, type IIIB and C injuries may be reconstructed with locoregional soft-tissue flaps, or may require free-tissue transfer.

The Byrd classification (13) focuses more on the energy of the injury mechanism and provides a more descriptive system for assessing associated soft-tissue damage. Type I injuries are from low-energy mechanisms and involve noncomminuted fractures with minimal soft-tissue damage. Type II injuries are caused by moderate-energy mechanisms and have larger skin lacerations and a broader zone of injury with skin and muscle contusion. Importantly, Type II injuries do not have devitalized muscle. Type III injuries are secondary to high-energy mechanisms and involve severely comminuted bone or bony defects, with extensive skin involvement and the presence of devitalized muscle. Finally, Type IV injuries are caused by extreme-energy mechanisms and include severe crush injuries, degloving, or vascular injury requiring repair for salvage.

Both of these systems are helpful for stratifying patients by injury severity and in aiding reconstructive planning. The Byrd classification more adequately describes the zone of injury and may prove more useful. For example, a Gustilo IIIC injury with arterial disruption may still be able to be reconstructed with a locoregional flap or even a skin graft over muscle. On the other hand, a Byrd IV injury can only be treated with free-tissue transfer, because, by definition, the local tissues are too involved in the zone of injury to be used for reconstruction.

Timing of Repair

Early, aggressive and serial debridement are the rule rather than the exception for lower extremity wounds (14). Contaminated, colonized, and devitalized tissue must be removed prior to reconstruction. Complete demarcation of the zone of injury usually occurs within the first few days after an injury.

Some authors have advocated the use of “emergency free-flaps” for reconstruction of complex wounds within the first 24 hours or following the first debridement (15). Arnez argues that meticulous debridement followed by immediate free-tissue transfer led to a higher flap success rate, shorter hospital stays, decreased overall cost, and shorter time to rehabilitation and weight bearing (15).

Byrd et al. (13) divided the postinjury period into three phases: the acute phase (first week), the subacute phase (1–6 weeks), where there is wound colonization with bacteria, and the chronic phase (more than 6 weeks), where the wound begins to granulate. They concluded that patients had far fewer complications when patients were treated with flap coverage when they were still in the acute—noncolonized—phase.

Patients who undergo a treatment delay have longer hospital stays, protracted rehabilitation, and longer times to bony union (16). The majority of authors suggest that coverage within the first five to seven days is preferred, but that treatment within the first two weeks—while suboptimal—can be acceptable (8,14).

Bone Reconstruction

Bony fixation is an important prerequisite to reconstruction. In a large percentage of patients, the most expeditious means of fixation is external pin fixation. In severe lower extremity wounds, the use of plates or intramedullary nails is precluded by the inability to provide adequate and stable soft-tissue coverage. Often, antibiotic bead spacers are placed in lieu of bone grafts and kept in place until grafting is undertaken.

Bone grafting is indicated for comminuted fractures or bony gaps less than approximately 10 cm. The timing of bone grafting is controversial. Some authors advocate early grafting at the time of initial flap coverage, but most advocate grafting after obtaining stable soft-tissue coverage (17).

Vascularized bone transfers are indicated for longer bony gaps. They can either be free or pedicled. Free transfer allows more degrees of freedom in reconstruction and allows harvest from the contralateral extremity. Vascularized bone transfers could theoretically be placed in the acute setting, but are not widely used (18). More frequently, definitive bony treatment is undertaken after soft-tissue coverage has been achieved.

The most useful and reliable flap for tibial reconstruction is the fibula; however, iliac crest, scapula, or even rib can be used (19). Iliac crest may be more useful for smaller defects and for reconstruction around the ankle (20). The flap can either be inset as a single piece, or may be "double-barreled" to provide a broader base of bone and improved stability. Prior to weight bearing, patients must wait until the bone has hypertrophied to avoid stress-fracturing of the graft. Hypertrophy often takes a prolonged time and the patients may require external support for 1.5 to 2 years (19), prior to being able to weight-bear on their own. Even after adequate hypertrophy, patients remain at risk for stress fracture.

Distraction osteogenesis—the Ilizarov procedure—may be used to bridge large bone gaps up to 12 cm (21). Heller and Levin (8) describe four methods of integrating the Ilizarov procedure into a reconstructive plan. The first involves acute placement of the Ilizarov to be used as an external fixator, with free-tissue transfer being used as a means of getting adequate soft-tissue coverage. The second is the use of the Ilizarov to correct secondary deformities in bone healing after conventional fixation and free-tissue transfer reconstruction of soft-tissue defects. The third is the use of the Ilizarov to regain bone length after acute limb shortening. By shortening the limb, the size of the soft-tissue defect may decrease enough to allow for a smaller flap to be used. The final method is classical distraction osteogenesis. With bone transport, not only is the bone generated of good quality and of the correct size, but also the soft tissues surrounding the defect are transported as well. This transport may preclude the need for free-tissue transfer.

Soft-Tissue Reconstruction

When considering options for soft-tissue reconstruction following trauma, one must first consider locoregional solutions. However, in severe injuries, the extent of the zone of injury often rules out the use of local or pedicled flaps. The choice of flap will depend on the factors previously mentioned: the size and type of tissue defect, the size of the zone of injury, and the necessary pedicle length. Flaps containing a significant muscular component are favored in lower extremity trauma, secondary to their ability to adequately fill dead space and provide tissues with good vascularity over the underlying bone (Figs. 1–3). The main flaps used are the latissimus

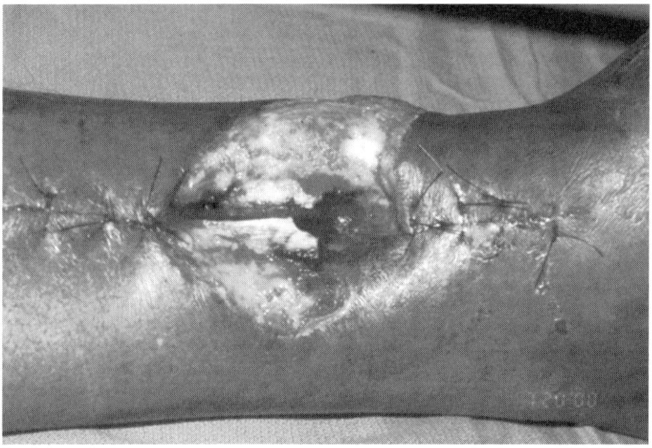

Figure 1 55-year-old male pedestrian struck by motor vehicle. Grade 3 open tibial fracture is shown.

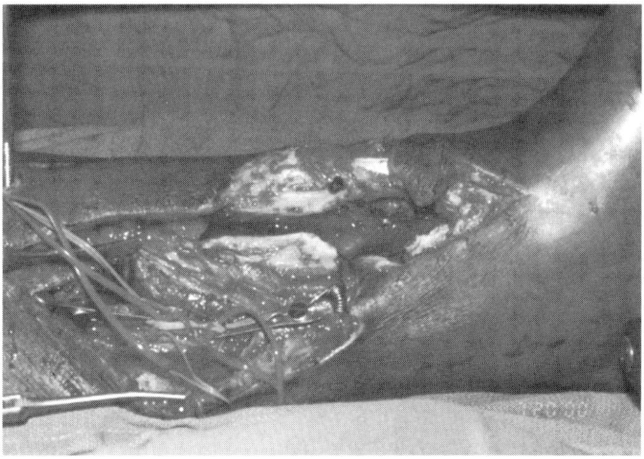

Figure 2 Exposure of posterior tibial vessels in preparation for microvascular transplant.

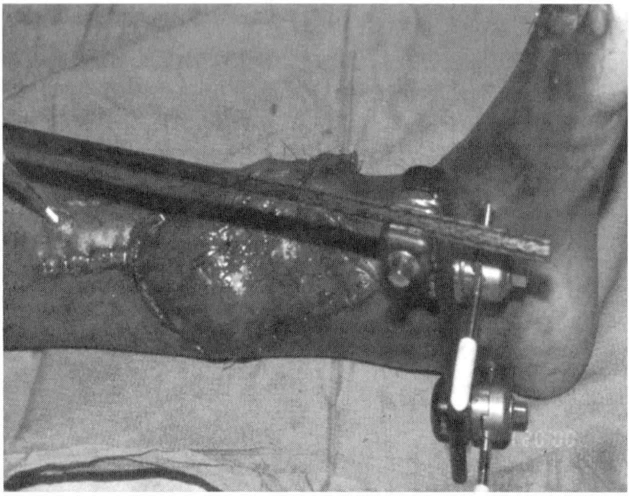

Figure 3 Rectus abdominis muscle transplant with skin graft to tibial defect.

dorsi, the rectus abdominis, the serratus anterior, and the gracilis. The anterolateral thigh flap can provide a large skin paddle, with minimal morbidity and without need to reposition the patient.

OSTEOMYELITIS

Treatment of chronic osteomyelitis involves aggressive debridement of infected, devitalized and compromised tissue, appropriate antibiotics, and obliteration of dead space. While local muscle flaps may work in some cases, often free-tissue transfer is necessary to completely fill the dead space created by sequestrectomy. Muscle flaps are preferred secondary to their bulk and their excellent vascularity. The free-flaps of choice are the same as are used to fill dead space after lower extremity trauma: the latissimus dorsi, the rectus abdominis, the serratus anterior, and the gracilis.

DIABETIC FOOT

Chronic ulcers in diabetic patients present a difficult treatment problem. Diabetic patients have poor healing and often have comorbidities, consequently having higher morbidity and more potential for mortality in the perioperative period (22). Patient selection, therefore, is of paramount importance. With proper patient selection, flap success rates can be equivalent to those in nondiabetic patients (5).

Free-tissue transfer has several advantages over locoregional flap reconstruction in the treatment of diabetic ulcers. First, the large amount of available tissue allows for aggressive debridement of the ulcer site and surrounding tissue. Second, the free-flap is well-perfused normal tissue that has good blood supply and which brings increased vascularization to the site of the wound.

ARTERIAL INSUFFICIENCY

Ulcers secondary to arterial insufficiency can be treated with free-tissue transfer. As with diabetic foot patients, dysvascular patients often have serious comorbidities, so patient selection is important. Prior to consideration of soft-tissue reconstruction, lower extremity revascularization should be undertaken. While some authors have proposed simultaneous revascularization and free-tissue transfer reconstruction (23), a more conservative approach may be preferable. Furthermore, functional outcomes must be high to justify the operative risk and use of resources.

POSTABLATIVE RECONSTRUCTION

The microsurgical armamentarium has facilitated limb salvage in patients following resection of neoplasms of the lower extremity. Distant free-tissue flaps bring healthy, nonradiated, well-perfused tissue into the ablative field. In addition to providing coverage, they allow restoration of contour and potentially recreation of load-bearing structures. Furthermore, increased vascularity helps wounds in radiated fields heal more effectively.

REFERENCES

1. Nichter LS, Morgan RF, Nichter MA. The impact of Indian methods for total nasal reconstruction. Clin Plast Surg 1983; 10(4):635–647.
2. Armstrong MB, Masri N, Venugopal R. Reconstructive microsurgery: reviewing the past, anticipating the future. Clin Plast Surg 2001; 28(4):671–673.
3. Kalderon AE. The evolution of microscope design from its invention to the present days. Am J Surg Pathol 1983; 7(1):95–102.
4. Jacobson J, Suarez E. Microsurgery in anastomosis of small vessels. Surg Forum 1960; 11:243–245.
5. Musharrafieh R, Saghieh S, Macari G, Atiyeh B. Diabetic foot salvage with microsurgical free-tissue transfer. Microsurgery 2003; 23(3):257–261.
6. Banic A, Wulff K. Latissimus dorsi free flaps for total repair of extensive lower leg injuries in children. Plast Reconstr Surg 1987; 79(5):769–775.
7. Ozkan O, Ozgentas HE, Islamoglu K, Boztug N, Bigat Z, Dikici MB. Experiences with microsurgical tissue transfers in elderly patients. Microsurgery 2005; 25(5):390–395.
8. Heller L, Levin LS. Lower extremity microsurgical reconstruction. Plast Reconstr Surg 2001; 108(4):1029–1041.
9. Park S, Han SH, Lee TJ. Algorithm for recipient vessel selection in free tissue transfer to the lower extremity. Plast Reconstr Surg 1999; 103(7):1937–1948.

10. Khouri RK, Shaw WW. Reconstruction of the lower extremity with microvascular free flaps: a 10-year experience with 304 consecutive cases. J Trauma 1989; 29(8):1086–1094.
11. Lange RH, Bach AW, Hansen, ST, Jr, Johansen KH. Open tibial fractures with associated vascular injuries: prognosis for limb salvage. J Trauma 1985; 25(3):203–208.
12. Gustilo RB, Mendoza RM, Williams DN. Problems in the management of type III (severe) open fractures: a new classification of type III open fractures. J Trauma 1984; 24(8):742–746.
13. Byrd HS, Spicer TE, Cierney G III. Management of open tibial fractures. Plast Reconstr Surg 1985; 76(5):719–730.
14. Celikoz B, Sengezer M, Isik S, et al. Subacute reconstruction of lower leg and foot defects due to high velocity-high energy injuries caused by gunshots, missiles, and land mines. Microsurgery 2005; 25(1):3–15.
15. Arnez ZM. Immediate reconstruction of the lower extremity—an update. Clin Plast Surg 1991; 18(3):449–457.
16. Godina M. Early microsurgical reconstruction of complex trauma of the extremities. Plast Reconstr Surg 1986; 78(3):285–292.
17. French B, Tornetta P. High-energy tibial shaft fractures. Orthop Clin North Am 2002; 33:211–230.
18. Tropet Y, Garbuio P, Obert L, Jeunet L, Elias B. One-stage emergency treatment of open grade IIIB tibial shaft fractures with bone loss. Ann Plast Surg 2001; 46(2):113–119.
19. Doi K, Akino T, Shigetomi M, et al. Vascularized bone allografts: review of current concepts. Microsurgery 1994; 15:831.
20. Hierner R, Wood M. Comparison of vascularized iliac crest and vascularized fibula transfer for reconstruction of segmental and partial bone defects in long bones of the lower extremity. Microsurgery 1995; 16(12):818–826.
21. Cierny G III, Zorn KE, Nahai F. Bony reconstruction in the lower extremity. Clin Plast Surg 1992; 19(4):905–916.
22. Ozkan O, Coskunfirat OK, Ozgentas HE. Reliability of free-flap coverage in diabetic foot ulcers. Microsurgery 2005; 25(2):107–112.
23. Lepantalo M, Tukiainen E. Combined vascular reconstruction and microvascular muscle flap transfer for salvage of ischaemic legs with major tissue loss and wound complications. Eur J Vasc Endovasc Surg 1996; 12(1):65–69.
24. Arnez ZM, Hanel DP. Free tissue transfer for reconstruction of traumatic limb injuries in children. Microsurgery 1991; 12(3):207–215.

8

Management of Lower Extremity Burn Injuries

Malachy E. Asuku
Department of Plastic and Reconstructive Surgery, Ahmadu Bello University Teaching Hospital, Kaduna, Nigeria

Robert L. McCauley
Department of Plastic and Reconstructive Surgery, Shriners Burns Hospital, Surgery and Pediatrics, University of Texas Medical Branch, Galveston, Texas, U.S.A.

ACUTE BURN INJURY

Burn injuries to the lower extremities are a major concern either as a result of a large total body surface area (TBSA) burn or as an isolated injury, especially to the foot (1,2). Such burn injuries can significantly affect the overall rehabilitation of the patient (1–5).

Lower extremity burns can result from a variety of agents occurring usually under accidental circumstances (2,3). While scald injuries and flame burns often result in superficial and deep partial thickness burns, contact burns and high-voltage electrical burns will often result in either full thickness burns or even fourth degree burns (4). Less common causes such as chemicals may also produce serious burns to the lower extremities (4). Aside from the depth of the burns, regional characteristics may have an impact on the severity of lower extremity burn injuries (1–6). Edema associated with deep partial and full thickness burn injury to the lower extremity can be made worse by dependency. Edema can also enhance inflammation, resulting in pain and a decrease in mobility of the injured parts. These circumstances can result in joint stiffness and may impair rehabilitation. In the acute phase of injury, control of edema is best accomplished by elevation of the affected part of the lower extremity. The goal of management is to facilitate early ambulation with compression garments (1,5,6).

Circumferential injuries resulting in edema in lower extremity burns can also lead to the development of a compartment syndrome. Elderly patients with peripheral vascular insufficiency and patients suffering high-voltage electrical injuries are reported to be at increased risk (1–3). A high index of suspicion is required to determine the need for immediate decompression (1–3). It is important to note that while peroneal nerve palsy may be due to direct injury to the common peroneal nerve at the neck of the fibular, it may also result from an impending compartment syndrome. Mani and Chhatre (1) insisted that escharotomies and fasciotomies when indicated should be done early in the resuscitative phase before tissue perfusion is compromised. Although the decision to decompress is often based on clinical features, effective tissue perfusion essentially stops when tissue pressure reaches 40 mmHg (1). Although escharotomy can be done at the bedside, fasciotomy requires more extensive preparation for anesthesia.

The involvement of the lower extremity in high-voltage electrical injuries also generates other concerns. The bulky muscles of the thigh may develop myonecrosis releasing large volumes of breakdown products that may constitute a significant threat to renal function (1). This danger, however, can be significantly minimized with diligent fluid therapy and timely debridement of nonviable muscle tissue. These patients may require additional reconstruction in order to close their wounds.

It is important to note that in lower extremity burns, there is a paucity of soft tissues over the tibial tuberosity, the shin, the malleoli, and the toes. Consequently, these areas are more predisposed to deep burns with exposure of tendons, bones, and joints. This is particularly evident following electrical burns (2,3). These areas may heal in a delayed fashion because they are devoid of the freely mobile soft-tissue padding required for any degree of wound contraction. Such areas may require the use of regional flaps or free tissue transfer in order to obtain satisfactory long-term results.

Often there is concern that lower extremity burn wounds may be at increased risk of wound infection since the perineum may be viewed as a potential source of contamination. This has led to the irrigation of the burned area rather than the immersion that is seen during tub room cleaning in some centers (1). Although this concern has remained unsubstantiated, meticulous wound care and appropriate bacterial monitoring should prevent the conversion of partial thickness wounds to deeper injuries. Superficial partial thickness burns are expected to heal with excellent functional and esthetic results within two weeks (1). On the other hand, deep partial thickness and full thickness burns require resurfacing with skin grafts or flaps. Unexpanded sheet grafts are preferred to mesh grafts in resurfacing the lower extremities. However, such an approach is subject to availability, whereas other areas such as the face and hands can take precedence (2,3).

Traditionally, the lower extremity constitutes the most frequently harvested donor site for autogenous skin grafts. The large and uniform surfaces provided by the thigh make it most suitable as a donor site. Therefore, when the thigh is involved in deep partial thickness or full thickness burns, one is not only faced with the problem of resurfacing a large area but also with the loss of a quality skin graft donor site. This, places a high premium on the availability of other donor sites. This is especially challenging when the injury is part of a large surface area burn. Under such circumstances, other less suitable donor sites such as the back, the buttocks, and the abdomen may have to be utilized. The use of skin substitutes, cultured autografts, and allografts in burns wound coverage must be seen as attempts to provide more options rather than as alternatives to autogenous skin grafts (1).

Ambulation following the application of skin grafts to the lower extremity at times has been controversial (7–12). However, early ambulation as soon as the grafts have "taken" securely should be the gold standard (6). The grafted lower extremity usually requires some type of compression garment during ambulation to minimize the effect of hydrostatic pressure and edema formation. The use of the Unna Boot® (Dome-Paste Bandage, Mile Inc., West Haven, Connecticut, U.S.A.) has been acclaimed to solve the problems of blistering and graft separation previously encountered with early ambulation (6,13,14).

Burns of the weight-bearing surface of the foot may be deep enough to require resurfacing in spite of the limited exposure of the area, the protection provided by the thickened epithelium, and the use of footwear. Such injuries are commonly encountered as exit wounds in electrical burns or arise from prolonged contact burns in patients with peripheral neuropathies (2,3,6,15,16). The main concern is to provide durable coverage. Destruction of the plantar fascia may disrupt the intrinsic mechanism of arch support and require long-term orthotic inserts (2,3). There are varied opinions as to the most suitable means of resurfacing the weight-bearing portion of the foot. Split thickness and full thickness skin grafts as well as pedicled flaps have all been utilized. However, each has fallen short of providing the highly specialized characteristics of the normal plantar skin (16–20). Kucan et al. (2,3) noted that a combination of flexibility and durability is required of any tissue used to resurface the sole of the foot. This must be accomplished without excessive tissue bulk that will accommodate the use of footwear. The requirement for ideal plantar resurfacing is therefore durable tissue of moderate volume that will affix tightly to deeper structures resisting shear forces and capable of attaining protective sensation. Kucan et al. also noted that split thickness skin grafts are no less durable than full thickness skin grafts. Consequently, split thickness skin grafts continue to be the primary method of coverage for the plantar surface as long as there is adequate supporting subcutaneous tissue.

Another area of concern following deep burns of the foot is the tendency to develop shortening of the Achilles tendon (6). Prompt and proper use of splints and casts may be required to maintain the ankle joint in a plantar-grade position while the proper use of footboards may suffice in the nonambulatory patient. However, careful monitoring of pressure points is required to prevent the development of pressure sores (6). The importance of maintaining joint motions particularly in the multijointed ankle and foot in the immediate postinjury period cannot be overemphasized. The biomechanics at these joints are highly complex with motions occurring simultaneously in a number of planes during both the weight-bearing and nonweight-bearing phases (2,3). Success at rehabilitation of the burned lower extremity will, therefore, depend on maintaining the function of these joints first and correction of any subsequent deformities second.

Finally, inpatient versus outpatient management of lower extremity burns has been debated. Zachary et al. (5) noted that isolated burns of the feet have the distinction of being the most common burn injury to be initially treated on an outpatient basis. Yet, many of these patients subsequently require hospitalization due to significant morbidity. They therefore suggested that patients with this injury are better served by inpatient care. Lyle et al. (15) in emphasizing the same view identified cellulitis, hypertrophied scarring, and prolonged hospitalization as possible complications of initial outpatient care of the burned foot. The American Burn Association concurs, recommending hospitalization for burns of the feet.

Although the depth of the injury is key to determining the complexity of treatment required in the acute care of the burned lower extremity, control of edema, early tangential excision and resurfacing with skin grafts, appropriate splinting, and early ambulation are fundamental rules to insure a successful outcome.

RECONSTRUCTION OF THE BURNED LOWER EXTREMITY

Although adequate acute care of lower extremity burns can significantly minimize the need for reconstructive procedures in later years, less than optimal outcomes may occur with deep injuries. The effects of weight bearing, as well as growth in patients who sustained early childhood burns, may also contribute to the development of deformities. Various reconstructive efforts may be required to maximize functional outcome of the thermally injured or deformed lower extremity. Brou et al. (21) noted that in a survey of 25 patients with a mean TBSA burn of 71% (65% full thickness), 27% (136/512) of the total reconstructive needs were in the torso and lower extremities. The principal reconstructive goals for the lower extremity are weight bearing and unimpeded ambulation. Achieving these goals requires stable, durable skin coverage with protective sensation. The final outcome should not only allow proper shoe fit but also play a role in boosting self-esteem and independence (2,3).

Experience has shown that the best way to meet the patient's goals is through an integrated team approach. According to Kucan et al. (2,3) reconstruction of the burned lower extremity may be divided into two phases: (i) early: beginning at admission and extending up to one year after injury; and (ii) late: commencing after one year of injury. In the early phase, reconstructive procedures may be required in the closure of complex wounds as well as in the prevention and correction of early onset functional impairments. The late phase, however, deals with problems of chronic instability of soft-tissue coverage, burn scar contractures, and contour deformities. In children, growth disturbances and revision of amputation stumps comes into play.

Early Reconstruction

Acute Wound Coverage

Reconstruction for acute wound coverage may be indicated in deep partial, full thickness, and fourth degree burns in which exposure of underlying structures may present significant wound coverage problems (2,3). These injuries commonly result from high-voltage electrical burns and contact burns characterized by muffler burns. Kucan et al. (2,3) observed that skin grafts are inadequate to achieve either short- or long-term reconstructive goals in these injuries. Invariably, composite tissues in the form of flaps are required for closure of such wounds, and options will depend on the size of the wound and its anatomical location.

The Thigh: The wide circumference of the thigh as well as the abundance of soft tissues allow for excision and primary closure of limited deep burn wounds. When soft-tissue loss is extensive, however, the first option lies in the use of adjacent soft tissues as advancement or transpositional flaps to close the defect. The nature as well as the location of the defect and recipient bed contributes to determining the tissues best suited for closure. Muscle flaps available for coverage of proximal wounds include the rectus abdominis, the tensor fascia lata, and the sartorius for smaller defects. In the formidable problem of deep burns of the groin with exposure of the external iliac and femoral vessels, closure requires bulky soft tissues to provide adequate padding and protection. The inferiorly based rectus abdominis muscle flap has been found useful in this reconstruction. More distal defects on the thigh have been reconstructed with the proximally based tensor fascia lata and the vastus medialis transposition muscle flaps (6,22). Salisbury and Bevin (22) suggested the use of the distally based sartorius muscle flap for coverage of defects of the distal thigh. They, however, recognize the need to determine the presence of the distal pedicle before clinical use.

Currently, the fasciocutaneous flap described by Ponsten in 1981 (23) and extensively applied to the management of burn injuries by Tolhurst et al. (24,25) in 1983 has become popular in the closure of deep burn wounds in the thigh. This flap allows a one-staged transfer without undue contour deformity and has the added advantage of not compromising functional muscle power (6). Barclay et al. as well as Cormack and Lamberty (26,27) described the blood supply to these flaps as arising through vessels that pass along the fascial septa between muscle bellies and then fan out at the level of the deep fascia to form a vascular plexus, which supplies the skin. The popliteal-posterior thigh fasciocutaneous flap introduced by Maruyama and Iwahira (28) in 1989, has also been described as a one-staged closure of deep burn wounds of the posteromedial and posterolateral thigh. This flap, which is distally based, is supplied by a direct branch of the popliteal artery that emerges through the fat between the semimembranous and biceps femoris at the level of the popliteal fossa. Preoperative angiography or Doppler flowmetry may be required to provide a safer outcome. The skin island is designed with its lateral margins situated between the hamstring muscles and can be raised proximally as far as the gluteal crease. The donor site may be closed primarily or require use of a split thickness skin graft (28). A similar distally based fasciocutaneous flap is the lower posterolateral thigh flap described by Laitung (29). The flap is supplied by the direct cutaneous branches of the popliteal artery and the lateral superior genicular artery and is also suitable for coverage of deep burn wounds of the anterolateral and posterior thigh (29).

The Knee: Deep burn injuries in the region of the distal thigh and upper leg can be compounded by involvement of the knee joint. When the joint space is exposed, immediate flap closure is required. Myocutaneous flaps and muscle flaps are well suited for such closures. Witt and Achauer noted that the advantages of myocutaneous flaps include their ability to obliterate dead spaces. At the same time, these flaps provide stable skin coverage and good blood supply that accelerates wound healing (6). However, the donor site deformity associated with the use of myocutaneous flaps has remained a major drawback. This issue is addressed in part in the use of muscle flaps with split thickness skin grafts as a single or staged procedure.

The gastrocnemius muscle provides by far the most versatile option in the closure of the opened knee joint. While the medial head can be designed to reach the anteromedial aspects of the knee joint, distal thigh and upper tibia, the lateral head is suitable for closures over the anterolateral aspect of the knee joint and upper tibia (30–32) (Fig. 1). The vascular supply to both heads are relatively consistent. Proximal exposure and separation of the two heads of the gastrocnemius muscle and identification of the soleus fascia are essential to distal separation and elevation of either of these flaps. The major disadvantages in the use of myocutaneous and muscle flaps include the sacrifice of functional muscle and the excessive bulk at the recipient site.

The popliteo-posterior thigh and the lower posterior-lateral thigh fasciocutaneous flaps have both been reportedly used in closure of such superficially opened knee joints. Microsurgical transfer of free flaps provides yet another option for closure of the opened knee joint. Although this option allows the one-stage use of high-quality distant tissues, it has been reserved for more severe cases in which the less complex local options are unavailable.

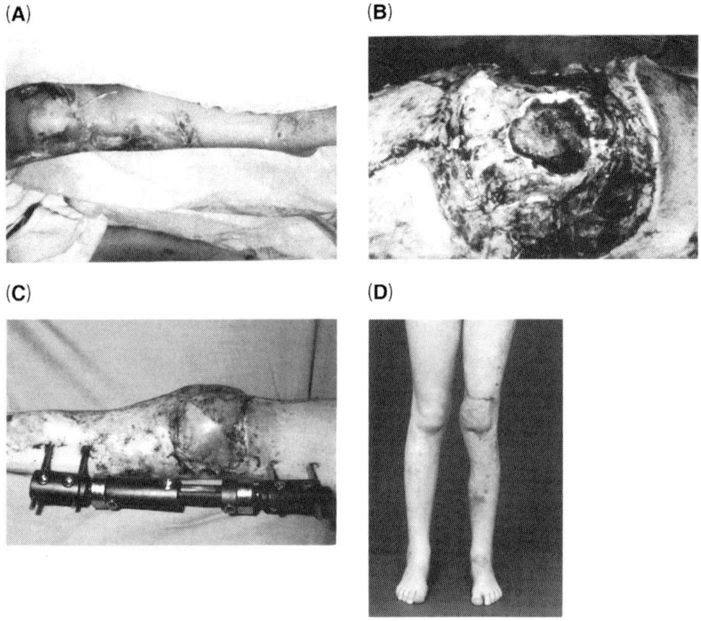

Figure 1 (A) Patient with full thickness burn over left knee after being trapped underneath a car with knee next to muffler. (B) Debridement showing open knee joint. (C) Medial gastronocnemius muscle flap for closure around the knee joint. (D) Final result after closure one year later. Source: From Ref. 33.

The Lower Leg: The closure of wounds in the distal part of the lower extremity is complex. Pedicled flaps in this region are sparse and small (2,3). Muscle flaps are the workhorses in the closure of deep burn wounds in this region. Sood et al. (34) observed that the superior third of the lower leg might be reliably covered with the gastrocnemius muscle while the soleus muscle provides a useful flap in the reconstruction of the middle third of the leg. Coverage of wounds in the distal third of the leg is more difficult with options limited to the use of the reversed soleus flap or free tissue transfer (34) (Fig. 2). Chang et al. and more recently Sood et al. (34,35) described the use of the tibialis anterior turnover muscle flap in the coverage of the exposed tibia following severe burns. This flap, which had previously been described for coverage of the tibia following trauma, provides good protection and blood supply to the underlying bone with minimal donor site morbidity (36–39) (Fig. 3).

The saphenous artery fasciocutaneous flap based on the distal continuation of the saphenous artery onto the lower leg provides a basis for a posteromedial flap, which can be used for closure of adjacent defects (40,41). Similarly, the superficial sural artery fasciocutaneous flap raised along the center of the posterior calf and as far distally as the Achilles tendon, can provide closure for

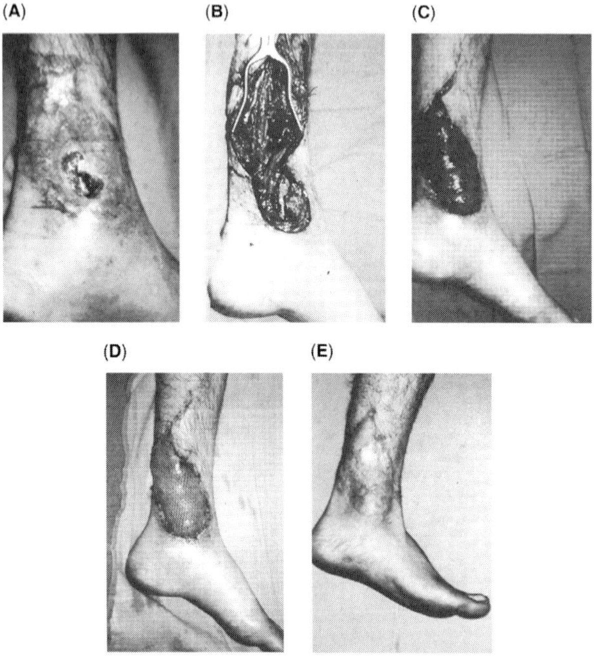

Figure 2 (**A**) Twenty-year-old male referred after motorcycle muffler burn over medial aspect of left ankle. Patient referred after failure of skin grafts for closure. (**B**) Patient noted to have osteomyelitis requiring extensive debridement of soft tissue and bone. (**C**) Coverage with a gracilis muscle flap. (**D**) Coverage of flap with a split thickness skin graft. (**E**) Appearance one year later after treatment of osteomyelitis with stable coverage and full weight bearing. *Source:* From Ref. 33.

adjacent burn wounds (41). Maruyama et al. (42) introduced the bilobed fasciocutaneous flaps for coverage of defects on the leg (Fig. 3). This is intended to improve donor site morbidity by avoiding the use of skin grafts. While this is a useful technique it may not be suitable for large burn wounds.

More recently, Heymans et al. (43) reported the use of the medial adipofascial flap of the leg for the coverage of full thickness burns exposing the tibial crest. The saphenous artery and the posterior tibial artery perforators constitute the blood supply of this flap, which can be mobilized to cover the whole length of the tibia. While the donor site is closed primarily, the flap requires coverage with split-thickness skin grafts. The old technique of shaving and overgrafting with thick split-thickness skin grafts to provide good skin protection over exposed tibia still has a place in the reconstruction of the severely burned leg. However, currently dermabrasion has replaced shaving of epithelial elements. In select cases, this technique may augment skin durability and obviate the need for flap reconstruction (44).

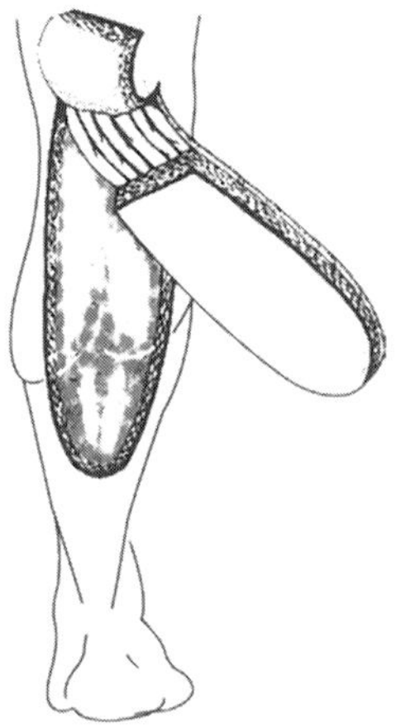

Figure 3 The island fasciocutaneous flap divided into two proximal random skin flaps will cover the popliteal region. The distal flap is transposed to cover the anterolateral part of the knee. Source: From Ref. 39.

Hammer et al. (45) as well as a number of other authors have reported satisfactory results with the use of the free latissimus dorsi flap in resurfacing the anterior surface of the lower leg in burned patients. The flap is broad, flat, and can be tailored to fit comfortably into most defects. Other free flaps suitable for resurfacing the burned lower leg include the rectus abdominis, serratus anterior, and the gracilis muscles covered with split-thickness skin grafts (3,6,46).

The Ankle and Achilles Tendon Areas: Closure of deep burn wounds in the ankle and Achilles tendon areas present special difficulties. Historically, the cross-leg fasciocutaneous flap provided the principal means of closure of such wounds (1). Today, the use of the thin local fasciocutaneous flaps has emerged. Masquelet et al. and Clark et al. (47,48) described the lateral supramalleolar fasciocutaneous flap based on the perforating branches of the peroneal artery. The flap is suitable for coverage of the distal Achilles tendon area and ankle defects. Several other similar lateral and posterior calf flaps based on the perforating vessels at the ankle and providing sensate coverage have been described. Their use in burn reconstruction may, however, be limited by the extent of the initial burn injury (49–51).

Microvascular free tissue transfers provide the most adequate means of resurfacing deep wounds in the ankle, malleolar, and Achilles tendon areas. The thinner fasciocutaneous and fascial free flaps are most suitable as they preserve the normal contour of the region. The radial forearm free flap, the medial and lateral arm flaps, the temporalis fascial flap, and the scapular flap have all been reported in the literature (3,52–56). These flaps provide satisfactory reconstruction so long as nonviable underlying bony prominences are adequately debrided or decorticated.

The Foot: Fourth degree burns to the foot may result from electrical injuries. Patients may present with exposed tendons, ligaments, and joint structures requiring early soft-tissue reconstruction. Frequently, distant flaps are required as the foot has scanty and relatively rigid soft tissues. The transfer of distant flaps to the foot was achieved by the cross-leg flap technique first introduced by Hamilton in 1854 (48). The technique, however, is cumbersome and requires multiple stages of surgery. It is associated with high morbidity and frequently results in less than optimal functional and esthetic outcome. It is not surprising that this technique has now been largely abandoned (3,26,57,58). Kucan et al., however, observed that the cross-leg flap might still be useful in certain rare instances. They suggested that the technique should be retained in the repertoire of the burn reconstructive surgeon (2,3).

Several thin cutaneous, myocutaneous, and fasciocutaneous regional flaps have since been introduced in the soft-tissue reconstruction around the foot. These include the extensor digitorum brevis myocutaneous flap, and the medial and lateral plantar fasciocutaneous flaps. But these flaps are of limited use in burn reconstruction where the injury may affect large and adjacent cutaneous areas (3,59–70). Consequently, the microsurgical transfer of distant tissues has become the gold standard in burn reconstruction around the foot when tendons or other deep structures are exposed. Free flaps have several advantages, including flexibility of design, shortened hospitalization, and decreased need for postoperative immobilization and physical therapy (2,3,6,71–73). The transfer of free muscle flaps resurfaced with split-thickness skin grafts has been acclaimed as most successful in reconstructing the sole of the foot and the heel (1–3,73). Kucan et al. (2,3) described the outcome as much more resistant over time to the shearing forces produced by walking. The free muscle flaps may look bulky initially, but they shrink over time due to the effect of denervation. This should obviate any need for early debulking (3). The latissimus dorsi muscle and myocutaneous free flaps seem to be the workhorse in lower extremity burn reconstruction (45,74–77). However, due to considerations for preservation of contour, the thinner fasciocutaneous and fascial free flaps have been widely used to resurface the dorsum of the foot. The commonly used flaps for this purpose include the radial forearm free flap, the medial and lateral arm flaps, the temporalis fascial flap, and even the omentum (3,52–56).

A major prerequisite in the use of free flaps is the availability of suitable recipient vessels in the vicinity of the wound or defect and yet outside the zone of injury. This requirement may not be readily met in the severely burned lower extremity. However, the concept of using uninjured extremities as free flap carriers to sites with inadequate local recipient vessels has addressed this concern to some extent (78–81). The contralateral limb, where suitable, has been used in lower extremity situations (82–86). In 1991, Lai et al. (82) reported the use of free latissimus dorsi muscle flap in the salvage of a limb that had suffered high-voltage electrical injury using the contralateral dorsalis pedis pedicle as recipient vessels. Similarly, Yamada et al. (83) in 1995 reported the use of the cross-leg free rectus abdominis muscle flap for lower limb reconstructions.

Early Reconstructive Issues

Hypertrophic Burn Scars: Hypertrophic scarring involving the foot may result in contour distortion severe enough to interfere with the use of footwear, impair ambulation, and affect bone growth (87). Isolated burns of the dorsum of the foot tend to result from scalds and grease burns, which may be associated with increased risk of hypertrophic scar formation (5). Furthermore, those resulting from flame burns often occur as part of larger surface area burns so that the burned foot receives attention only after life-threatening issues and higher-priority areas have been addressed (5). Deitch et al. (88) noted that a major functional and esthetic problem in patients surviving thermal injuries is the development of hypertrophic burn scars. They noted that an important factor in the development of hypertrophic scarring is the time required for the burn wound to heal. In a series of 100 patients, they observed hypertrophic scarring in 33% of burn sites when the wound healed between 14 and 21 days and 78% of burn sites that healed after 21 days.

Larson et al. in 1971 popularized the use of pressure garments in the control and prevention of hypertrophic burn scars (89–91). Although this concept later was met with controversy, it has remained an adjunct in the control of burn scars. The requirements include the provision of continuous pressure of the magnitude of 25 mmHg above the capillary pressure and long-term use of the garments usually for several months. Frequent careful evaluation is necessary to ensure the effectiveness of the program. Hypertrophic scars are believed to be most responsive to pressure therapy in the first three to six months when they are immature, soft, and often tender. Silicone gel inserts were later found to be equally effective in controlling and preventing the development of hypertrophic burn scars (92). Silicone gel was further reported to soften the matured hypertrophic scar and to decrease shrinkage and contraction of healed skin grafts. Although the mode of action of silicone gel is yet to be completely understood, it certainly does not depend on pressure (92).

Surgical correction is often required for hypertrophic burn scars if function or cosmesis is affected. Focal and linear hypertrophic scars of an unfavorable nature can be excised and the wound primarily closed. However, the broad and unsightly hypertrophic scars with fissures and recurrent cellulitis may be better served by surgical excision and resurfacing with thick split-thickness or full-thickness skin grafts.

Early Burn Scar Contractures: Burn wounds have been shown to exhibit exaggerated wound contraction during healing. The contraction has also been shown to persist within the burn scar tissue particularly where the scar has remained active and hypertrophic (89–91). Over the flexor surfaces of joints, the force of wound contraction may act with contraction of the underlying flexor muscles, resulting in the development of contractures (89–91). While early mild to moderate contractures may respond to physical therapy programs, the severe and longstanding contractures invariably require surgical release. Physical therapy programs for early, less severe contractures include range of motion exercises and the use of static and dynamic splints (89–91,93–95). Several investigators observed that a fraction of those that fail to respond to these traditional approaches may respond to serial casting (93,94). This approach stretches the muscle, tendon, and joint capsules and gradually restores joint function. Splints may be required at the end of the serial casting to maintain the achieved correction. Serial casting is particularly useful in the pediatric age group because the success of the technique does not depend significantly on the patient's cooperation (93,94). Bennett et al. (93), however, noted that serial casting is mostly successful in large joints with fewer planes of motion and large lever arms.

Dorsal contractures of the foot are unlikely to respond to conservative measures. Surgical intervention is reserved for those deformities, which are likely to be unresponsive to conservative measures. Early surgical intervention may be required if the incapacitating late complication of the rocker-bottom deformity is to be avoided (2,3). The quality of the overlying soft-tissue scar determines whether a simple incisional release or complete excision and resurfacing is required. Resurfacing with thick split-thickness or full-thickness skin grafts will usually suffice. However, when this is less than optimal, flap coverage must be provided. The physical therapy with splints and range of motion exercises as well as the use of custom-made padded shoes with rigid soles are essentials to obtaining satisfactory outcome. Although some authors have cautioned against surgery on immature burn scars and contractures on the grounds of high recurrence rates, there are instances when progressive functional impairment may be better served by early surgical intervention (95,96).

Late Reconstruction

Unstable Scars

A potential problem with burn injuries is the development of poor-quality wound healing by secondary intention. This may result in unstable scars capable of interfering with hygiene and function. Spontaneous healing following deep second-degree burns results in unstable coverage that is prone to recurrent ulcerations and hypertrophic scarring. The resurfacing of the burned lower extremity with split-thickness skin grafts meshed to a ratio greater than 1:2 may also contribute to subsequent scar instability (90).

Chronic ulcerations and unstable scars tend to occur also in relation to contractures where countermovement is retained and in areas prone to repetitive trauma (2,3). Such areas in the lower extremity include the anterior aspect of the knee joint, the popliteal area, the anterior aspect of the ankle joint, the malleolar and Achilles tendon areas, and the dorsal surfaces of the toes. Under normal circumstances, these areas are provided with thin, pliable skin overlying scanty subcutaneous tissues. In the severely burned lower extremity, however, unyielding scars and skin grafts may be incapable of withstanding the tension created in the region. Furthermore, in the region of the foot, skin grafts may fail to provide the required durability to withstand the stress and strain of constant contact with footwear and ambulation. Kucan et al.(2,3) noted that split-thickness skin graft coverage of the foot may result in hyperkeratosis along the junction of the graft and surrounding skin, fissure formation, ulceration, breakdown and the development of burn scar contractures. They, however, suggested that split-thickness grafts may be used in early coverage to give the patient and surgeon added time to develop a more adequate reconstructive plan.

Chronic ulcerations are often painful. They can be complicated by excessive damage leading to further discomfort in the rehabilitation of the burned patient (90). Unstable scars can also delay the onset of physical therapy by inhibiting the use of splints and pressure garments. This, in effect, may protract the course of overall rehabilitation. The goal of management in patients with unstable scars and chronic ulcers is to obtain stable and durable soft-tissue coverage. Complete excision or dermabrasion of the poor-quality skin and resurfacing with thick split-thickness or full-thickness sheet grafts will usually give satisfactory results. Achauer and Vanderkam described the unstable burn scar of the anterior knee as a primary reconstructive problem in which coverage with skin grafts may be too thin, leading to unstable correction (95). They advocated overgrafting with a medium to thick split-thickness skin graft or even with a full-thickness graft. While this may suffice in the adult, it may not provide the long-term stable coverage required in the growing child (97). Dhanraj et al. (98), in a review of the management of recalcitrant knee ulcers in pediatric patients, observed that excessive longitudinal tension played a contributory role in the etiology of the ulcers. They demonstrated permanent closure of the ulcers when the tension in the lower thigh was eliminated by transverse incisional release and resurfacing with wide sheet split-thickness skin grafts (Fig. 4).

(A) (B) (C)

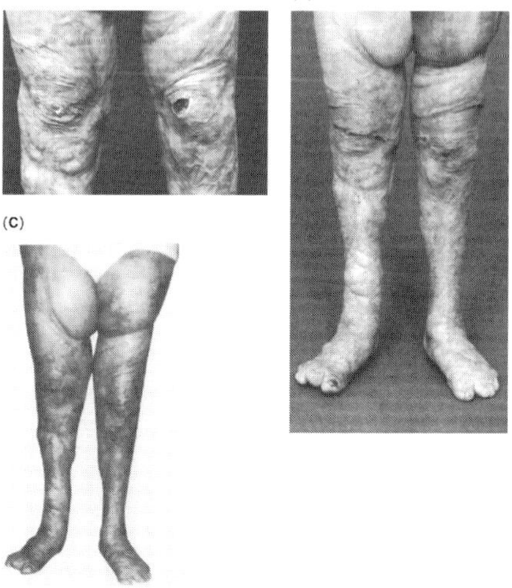

Figure 4 (**A**) Eleven-year-old male with bilateral recalcitrant knee ulcers. He had suffered 62% TBSA burns at the age of one and has had a total of three previous ulcer excisions and grafting to both knees. (**B**) Four weeks postincisional release and grafting of 160 cm^2 of split thickness skin graft to the left thigh and 120 cm^2 to the right. Both ulcers completely closed. (**C**) Patient remained ulcer free at two years' follow-up. *Abbreviation:* TBSA, total body surface area. *Source:* From Ref. 98.

Kucan et al. (2,3) observed that the unique architecture of the skin and subcutaneous tissues of the sole of the foot is specifically adapted for weight bearing and cannot be satisfactorily reproduced by available reconstructive techniques. They noted that distant flaps of nonglabrous skin used to resurface the sole of the foot lack the fibrous elements that bind the normal sole to the underlying tissues. The transferred tissue is, therefore, unstable over the underlying bony skeleton and is unable to resist the shear forces during ambulation. In a recent survey of various techniques available for the reconstruction of the sole of the foot, it was noted that the overall incidence of chronic ulceration in fasciocutaneous flaps and skin grafted muscle flaps did not differ significantly. Furthermore, flap sensibility was not different using the two techniques (2,3). The inference, therefore, is that these chronic ulcers are mechanical in origin. They occur either from untreated osseous abnormalities or from external friction due to poor-fitting footwear (2,3). Meticulous attention to contours while resurfacing the foot should reduce the problems of shoe fit and frictional ulcers. Kucan et al. (2,3) observed that aside from patient selection and postoperative education on the care of the reconstructed foot, the use of custom-made orthotics and padded shoes based on computer-assisted gait analysis are additional factors that enhance long-term successes.

Postburn unstable scars and chronic ulcers in the lower extremity deserve prompt attention particularly, having been shown to exhibit an increased risk of malignant transformation. The malignancy, which is described as Marjolin's ulcer, is a squamous cell carcinoma (1,99–103). The exact incidence of malignant degeneration in burn scars is not known; however, it has been estimated that up to 2 percent of all epidermoid carcinomas of the skin originate in burn scars (99). Several investigators observed a definite predilection for the flexion creases of the extremities (99–101). A latent period of several years to decades of chronic ulcerations in the burn scar may precede malignant degeneration (99–102).

Burn Scar Contractures

Burn scar contractures are a common and frustrating sequelae of thermal injury (89–91). The depth of the initial injury contributes in no small measure to the development of contractures. In the lower extremities, factors contributing to the development of postburn contractures include prolonged immobilization and inadequate skin coverage. Additionally, poor compliance with physical therapy programs aimed at minimizing scar hypertrophy and contractures may play a significant role. Larson et al. noted that the burn wound has an inherent tendency to contract and continues to do so until it meets an opposing force (89–91). They also stated that the position of comfort is the position of deformity, and that the severity of the deformity may be directly related to the depth of the initial injury (89–91,96). Robson et al. (96) observed that splinting and exercise are important means of providing the required opposing force to halt the development of contractures. Late, established contractures require surgical intervention. Peacock et al. (104) observed that the need for secondary reconstructive procedures following burn injuries is decreased by the proper attention to positioning and ranging of joints during the acute phase. They further stated that the success rates of such procedures increase in direct proportion to the degree of motion preserved in these joints before reconstruction.

Contractures of the Hip Joint: Hip contractures may result from deep burns of the anterior aspect of the upper thigh, the groin, and lower abdomen in children or from poor compliance with an established physical therapy program. The flexion contracture is usually accompanied by some degree of adduction as a result of the slight internal rotation that occurs with flexion at the hip joints. Surgical release may be indicated in all but the very mild and early contractures where splinting and positioning may constitute adequate treatment. The Z-plasty and its modifications as well as other local transposition flaps may be effective in breaking up and correcting contractures resulting from narrow restricting bands. However, the contractures frequently encountered are broad and may require more elaborate procedures for correction (105). The contracture is released with an incision parallel to the inguinal ligament through the breadth and thickness of the scarred tissue. The resulting defect is resurfaced with thick split-thickness or full-thickness skin grafts depending on availability and surgeon preference. Immobilization in extension is essential in the immediate postoperative period. Range of motion exercises as well as ambulation should be instituted as soon as the skin grafts take satisfactorily and stability is achieved. The proponents of flap coverage argue that such difficulties with the use of skin grafts might have contributed to the initial development of the groin contracture (105,106). However, the recent introduction of the vacuum-assisted closure technique to improve graft take in difficult contour areas such as the groin may address some of these concerns (107–110).

Flap coverage becomes an absolute necessity in case of exposure of the femoral vessels and nerve during the release of severe groin contractures (105). The large fasciocutaneous flaps popularized by Ponsten in 1981 have been used in these cases (Fig. 5) (23). Described as the "super-flap," the fasciocutaneous flaps are easy and quick to raise, can tolerate a length-breadth ratio of four-to-one, and donor defects can usually be closed directly. The flap can be raised in scarred or grafted skin, and yet survive transposition due to its fascial component (105,106). Turley et al. (105) reported the use of the medial fasciocutaneous flap of the thigh for release of postburn groin contractures. They obtained satisfactory outcome in their series that consisted of four patients with six severe groin contractures. The vascular supply and innervation of the flap had previously been described by Wang et al. (111) who used the same flap laterally for groin reconstruction and medially for vaginal and perineal reconstructions. Another option, which may be less versatile for the release of groin contractures, is the anteromedial thigh fasciocutaneous flap described by Hayashi and Maruyama in 1988 (112). The perfusion of this flap, like the medial thigh flap, is nonaxial and is dependent on the extensive vascular communications between the suprafascial and subdermal plexus of the thigh (113).

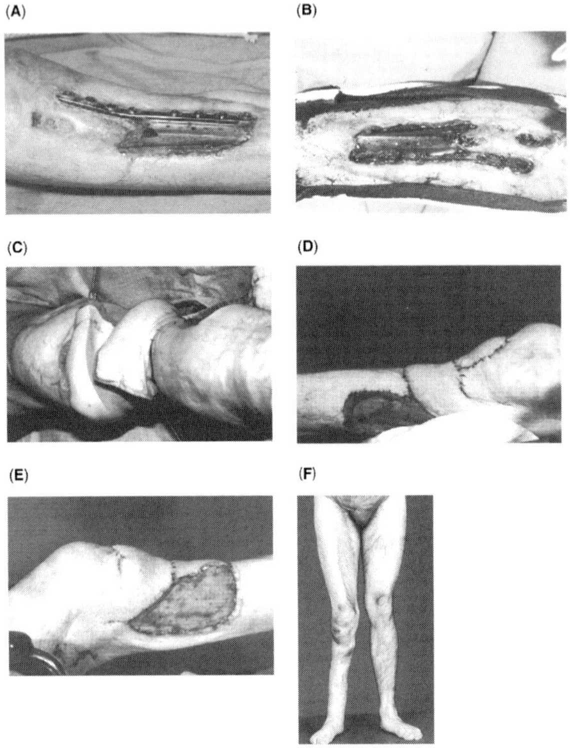

Figure 5 (**A**) Twelve-year-old male referred after motor vehicle accident where he sustained an open tibial fracture and arterial repair (femoral-popliteal bypass) to the right lower leg with exposed hardware. (**B**) Hardware removed and wound subsequently debrided. (**C**) Bilateral fasciocutaneous flaps used to cover the defect over the proximal lower leg. (**D**) Medial view of flaps and skin grafts used to cover the donor site. (**E**) Lateral view of flaps and skin grafts used to cover the donor site. (**F**) Eight-year follow-up with stable wound coverage. *Source:* From Ref. 33.

On occasion, the relatively bulky muscle and myocutaneous flaps may better serve the defect resulting from the release of groin contractures. The tensor fascia latae, rectus abdominis, gracilis, and sartorius muscles have been used either as muscle flaps or myocutaneous flaps in such circumstances (114,115). Turley et al. (105) noted that the use of flaps obviates the need for prolonged splinting.

Popliteal Contractures: Postburn flexion contractures of the knee joint, also known as popliteal contractures, are perhaps the most frequently encountered in the lower extremity. Yet, they are easily preventable (1). Early surgical intervention as well as early and aggressive physical therapy programs should serve to prevent and reduce the incidence of these contractures. Treatment options for popliteal contractures may correlate with the severity of the contracture as it affects limb function. Incisional or excisional release and skin grafting is frequently the first line of therapy with excellent long-term results. Fasciocutaneous and fascial flaps, which are devoid of bulk, may be used as alternatives. Prakash et al. (116) introduced the concept of the central segment expansion method in the release of severe popliteal burn scar contractures. The technique involves making releasing incisions proximal and distal to the level of the joint, thereby creating a bipedicle flap over the joint. The defects on either side of the flap are then covered with split-thickness skin grafts. Contraction of the split-thickness skin grafts is expected to result in the slow expansion of the flap.

Extensive contractures may require multiple incisions and therefore multiple bipedicle flaps sandwiched between skin grafts. Some authors advocated excision and coverage with the superiorly based medial or lateral fasciocutaneous flap in the presence of unstable scars or chronic ulcers. They, however, extended the concept of flap expansion by using narrow flaps such that defects above and below the flap are again resurfaced with skin grafts (117). The disadvantage of this approach however, is that it is staged, protracted and yet to be supported by any long-term follow-up results. More recently, however, Prakash et al. (118) reported the use of the posterior calf fascial flap in resurfacing popliteal defects after excision of contractures with unstable scars. They noted that the advantages of the technique include its reliability, since the strong fascia ensures satisfactory graft take, thereby preventing recurrence of the contracture. They also noted that harvesting the fascial flap is associated with no functional loss and minimal donor site defect. Robert et al. (119) had previously described the use of the same flap in the reconstruction of traumatic lower extremity defects.

Severe contractures, such as fixed flexion contractures, may require more complex reconstructive efforts. The potential problems include shortening and bow stringing of the hamstring tendons, the neurovascular bundles, and anterior dislocation of the knee. There is a need for a large amount of soft tissue for coverage when the contracted structures are released. The goal is to obtain satisfactory extension without compromising the perfusion and sensibility of the distal limb (120). Ahmad et al. (120) reported the use of Z-lengthening of contracted hamstring tendons and coverage with the medial gastrocnemius muscle flap. They resorted to the use of additional turnover adipofascial flap to cover residual lateral defects in one of the very severe cases in their series of five patients with seven severe popliteal contractures. They emphasized the need for postoperative splinting in plaster cast, followed by regular physiotherapy and use of pressure garments in order to achieve complete extension with full range of motion. The presence of bony ankylosis is an indication for osteotomy to remove the bridging bone and restore joint motion. Supracondylar extension osteotomy of the femur has been reported for correction of severe contractures in patients with neurological deficits such as myelomeningocele and cerebral palsy. However, this has not been reported in the correction of postburn contracture deformity (120,121).

Contractures of the Ankle Joint: The postburn contractures encountered at the ankle joint are either in dorsiflexion or in plantarflexion. The dorsiflexion contracture results from deep dorsal burns and usually occurs in concert with extension contractures of the toes due to involvement of the dorsum of the forefoot.

Transverse incisional release and resurfacing the defect with thick split-thickness or full-thickness skin grafts may be all that is required. Postoperative immobilization in a slightly overcorrected position is encouraged. Early range of motion exercises as well as use of pressure garments are essential in the restoration of form and function. Correction of severe contractures requires the excision of dense contracted scar, which may result in extensive soft-tissue defects and exposure of the extensor tendons. Adequate release may require tenolysis, tenotomies, capsulotomies, and even osteotomies (122). Joint stabilization with Kirschner's wires or insertion of Steinman pins for subsequent skeletal traction may also be required. Following such extensive release procedures, the defect may be resurfaced with thick split-thickness or full-thickness skin grafts (Fig. 6). However, where these are inadequate, flap coverage will be required. Local fasciocutaneous flap such as the lateral supramalleolar fasciocutaneous flap based on the perforating branches of the peroneal artery is a suitable option if available (47,48). However, microsurgical transfer of distant tissues offers the most attractive option in this region. The free radial forearm fasciocutaneous flap, the lateral arm fasciocutaneous flap, and the free temporoparietal fascial flap covered with

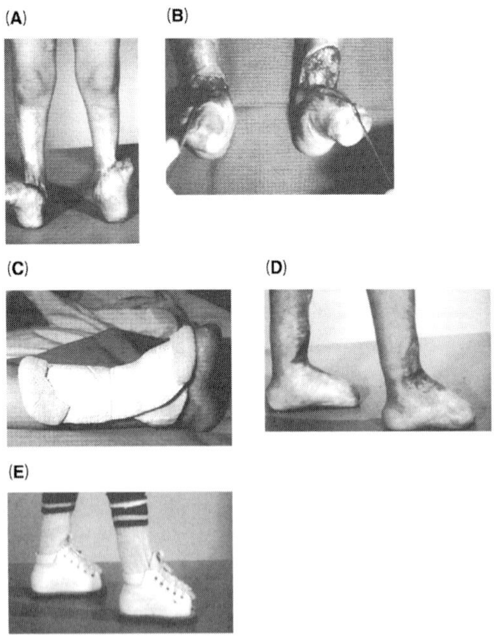

Figure 6 (**A**) Two-year-old child referred after severe burns to the lower extremities, which were allowed to heal by secondary intention. (**B**) Bilateral release performed with resurfacing with thick split-thickness skin grafts. (**C**) Both feet were splinted after graft take. (**D**) Three months later both feet in neutral position. (**E**) Patient shown in first pair of shoes.

split skin graft have been used extensively in this reconstruction where contour preservation is a major concern (52,123,124).

The less common plantarflexion contractures at the ankle joint are commonly due to Achilles tendon shortening. Achilles tendon shortening is a ubiquitous problem in the extensively burned patient with lower extremity involvement (6,94). Uncorrected, the progressive shortening is capable of resulting in the equinus deformity in which the musculoskeletal structures of the forefoot are secondarily deformed. Surgical correction is directed at tendon lengthening and the more difficult problem of providing suitable coverage. Options for tendon lengthening include the Z-lengthening and skin-strip lengthening techniques. Ideal coverage should provide adequate soft-tissue padding to allow healing and subsequent gliding of the tendon. Yet, it must be thin enough to preserve the normal contour of the area in order to permit use of normal footwear (1,6). Local flaps capable of meeting these requirements are difficult to come by. The lateral supramalleolar fasciocutaneous flap has been used for this purpose but again it may not be available in the severely burned lower extremity. Other local flaps that have been used include the inferiorly based de-epithelized turnover flap covered with a split skin graft described by Ramakrishnan et al. in 1985 (125). They reported a series of 35 patients in whom the use of this flap provided satisfactory long-term coverage of the Achilles tendon area (125). Microsurgical techniques have also allowed satisfactory coverage of these defects with high-quality distant tissues. The free fasciocutaneous and fascial flaps are particularly favored to preserve the desired contour. Chicarilli et al. (55) reported the use of a free radial forearm flap in resurfacing the Achilles tendon area utilizing the posterior tibial vessels as recipient vessels. They stated that the flap provided a thin, well-vascularized cutaneous restoration with a satisfactory esthetic result and low complication rate.

Contractures of the Forefoot: Deep burns of the dorsum of the forefoot frequently result in simple extension contractures of the toes. More severe and extensive dorsal burns, however, may produce the debilitating deformity in which the toes are hyperextended with subluxation or dislocation of the metatarsophalangeal joint. There may be associated loss of the transverse arch resulting in interdigital contractures with overriding of the toes. This deformity may interfere with normal weight bearing and ambulation leading to gait abnormalities. Pap et al. observed that burns of the feet could result in significant morbidity with protracted convalescence and extended absence from work and school (126). They, therefore, advocated that this injury should be given relatively high priority in all phases of care. The reconstructive goal is to restore normal anatomy that will permit unimpeded weight bearing and ambulation as well as allow the use of normal footwear (2,3).

While mild to moderate linear burn scar contractures of the dorsum of the foot may be corrected with Z-plasties and other local transposition flaps, the majority of the cases exhibit extensive soft-tissue deficiency requiring release and replacement with skin grafts or flaps. The deficiency of soft tissue in the long axis of the foot is frequently addressed by a transverse releasing incision over all metatarsophalangeal joints (15). On rare occasions, release of severe contractures may require tenotomies of the long extensors and capsulotomies of the metatarsophalangeal joints (1). Intermedullary bone fixation with Kirschner wires may be required to maintain joint position. Resurfacing with thick split-thickness or full-thickness skin grafts will usually suffice. Waymack et al. (87) reported a 15% recurrence rate within four years in a series of 55 children who had 90 reconstructive procedures for the treatment of early burn scar contractures of the feet. They stated that the recurrence rate was influenced by compliance with postoperative splinting rather than the use of either full thickness or split thickness skin grafts. Alison et al. (4), however, observed that the high recurrence rate following release of foot contractures might be related to the concomitant soft-tissue deficiency in the transverse metatarsal arch that is often unaddressed (Figs. 7 and 8). In a comparative analysis, Alison et al. (4) observed that the overall recurrence rate in their series of 68 children who had a total of 146 releases for foot contractures was 35.7% when only the longitudinal arch was released. The time interval before recurrence averaged 3.50 ± 0.41 years. However, with the additional release of the transverse arch, the time interval before recurrence averaged 4.29 ± 1.27 years. With improvements in execution of the technique, they subsequently recorded no recurrences. The group also believed that recurrence was influenced by the expansion ratio of the meshed split-thickness skin grafts used for coverage in the acute phase of management (4). They found that the time interval between injury and the need for the first surgical release when expansions of 1:2 were used doubled the interval recorded in the use of expansions of 1:4.

Dhanraj et al. (127) documented the efficacy of simultaneous bilateral surgical correction over staged sequential correction of burn scar extension contractures of the foot in patients with bilateral deformities. They noted that

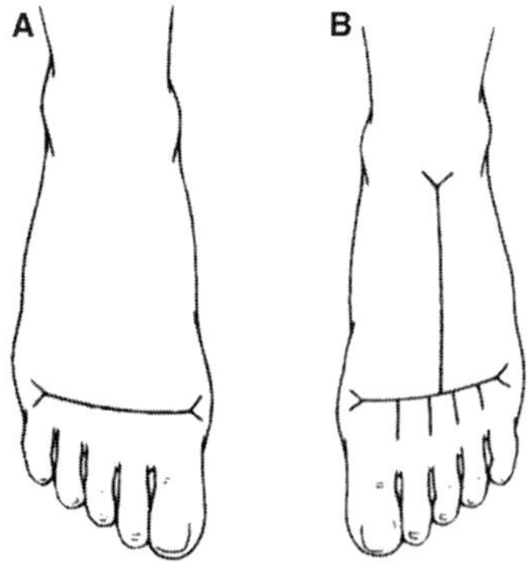

Figure 7 (**A**) Surgical release of the longitudinal metatarsal arch by a perpendicular incision over the metatarsal phalangeal joints. (**B**) Combined surgical release of both the longitudinal and transverse metatarsal arches. Additional incisions are parallel to the plane of the metatarsals. *Source:* From Ref. 4.

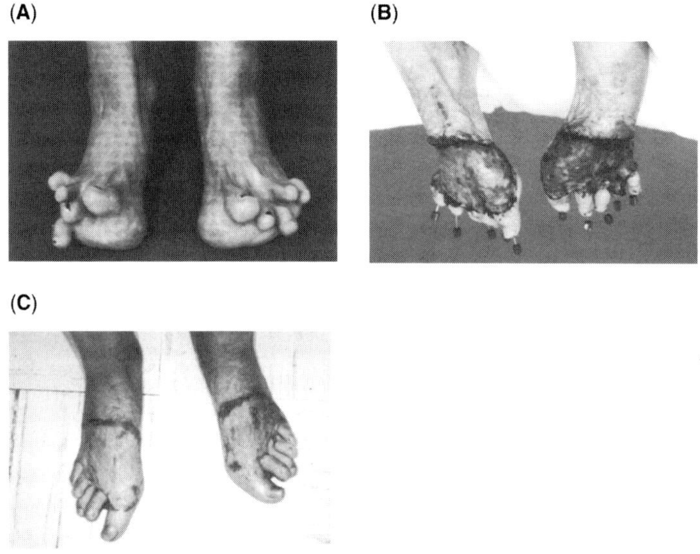

Figure 8 (**A**) Thirteen-year-old female referred for reconstruction of her feet: note severe subluxative at the metatarsal joints and loss of the transverse and longitudinal arches of the feet. (**B**) Correction with split thickness skin grafts and K-wire fixature pins left in place for six weeks. (**C**) Three-month follow-up.

there is no difference in morbidity or length of hospital stay between unilateral versus simultaneous bilateral correction with Kirschner wire fixation.

Web space contractures of the toes may accompany both dorsal burns and plantar burns. The associated functional impairment is usually minimal as a result of which surgical correction is rarely undertaken. However, esthetic concerns as well as repeated fungal infection may compel a patient to request surgical correction. The Z-plasty and its modifications as well as the V–M and the Y–V transposition flaps are favored because they obviate the need for skin grafts (1,6,15).

Flexion contractures of the toes frequently follow deep burns of the plantar surface of the foot. The contractures can be corrected by incisional release and resurfacing with split-thickness skin grafts. Postoperative immobilization is, however, difficult and may be accomplished by the use of intermedullary Kirschner wires in severe cases. Maintenance of the release requires the wearing of shoes with custom-made inserts to prevent recontracture (6). Achauer et al. (6), however, observed that the correction of these contractures with a variety of local flaps fashioned from the lateral aspect of the toes tend to produce more rapid healing and a more lasting correction. Care must, however, be taken not to compromise weight-bearing surfaces while using such local flaps.

The reconstructive plan for the correction of the multiple deformities that may arise from severe burns of the foot must be based on accurate evaluation and

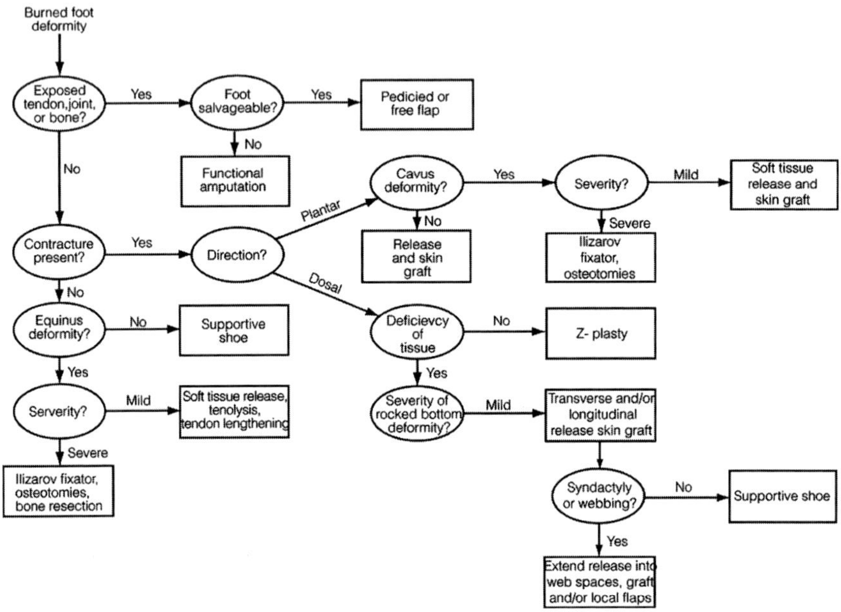

Figure 9 Algorithm for reconstruction of the burned foot. *Source*: From Ref. 15.

due considerations of the available reconstructive options suited to the individual patient (Fig. 9). In severe deformities early consultation should help in the formulation of a reconstructive timetable. The role of an adequate physical therapy program in the overall rehabilitation of the patient cannot be overemphasized.

REFERENCES

1. Mani MM, Chhatre M. Reconstruction of the burned lower extremity. Clin Plast Surg 1992; 19(3):693–703.
2. Kucan JO, Bash D. Reconstruction of the burned foot. Clin Plast Surg 1992; 19(3):705–719.
3. Goldberg DP, Kucan JO, Bash D. Reconstruction of the burned foot. Clin Plast Surg 2000; 27(1):145–161.
4. Alison WE, Moore ML, Reilly DA, et al. Reconstruction of foot burn contracture in children. J Burn Care Rehabil 1993; 14:34–38.
5. Zachary LS, Heggers JP, Robson MC, et al. Burns of the feet. J Burn Care Rehabil 1987; 8(3):192–194.
6. Witt PD, Achauer BM. Lower extremity. In: Achauer BM, ed. Burn Reconstruction. New York: Thieme Medical Publishers, 1991.
7. Schmitt MA, French L, Kalil PT. How soon is safe? Ambulation of the patient with burns after lower extremity skin grafting. J Burn Care Rehabil 1991; 12:33–37.

8. Bodenham DC, Watson R. The early ambulation of patients with lower limb grafts. Br J Plast Surg 1971; 24:20–22.
9. Johnson CL. Ambulating patients after lower extremity grafting. J Burn Care Rehabil 1984; 5:114–115.
10. Burnsworth B, Krob MJ, Langer-Schnepp M. Immediate ambulation of patients with lower extremity grafts. J Burn Care Rehabil 1992; 13:89–92.
11. Golden PT, Power CG, Skinner JR, et al. A technique of lower extremity mesh grafting with early ambulation. Am J Surg 1977; 133:646–647.
12. Sharpe D, Cardoso E, Baheti V. The immediate mobilization of patients with lower limb skin grafts: a clinical report. Br J Plast Surg 1983; 36:105–108.
13. Cox GW, Griswold JA. Outpatient skin grafting of extremity burn wounds with the use of Unna Boot(compression dressings. J Burn Care Rehabil 1993; 14:455–457.
14. Harnar T, Engrav LH, Marvin J, et al. Dr Paul Unna's boot and early ambulation after skin grafting the leg: a survey of burn centers and a report of twenty cases. Plast Reconstr Surg 1982; 69:359–360.
15. Lyle WG, Phillips LG, Robson MC. Reconstruction of the foot. In: Herndon DN, ed. Total Burn Care. Philadelphia: WB Saunders,1996:515–519.
16. Heimburger RA, Marten E, Larson DL, et al. Burned feet in children, acute and reconstructive care. Am J Surg 1973; 125:575–579.
17. Brown JB, Cannon B. The repair of surface defects of the foot. Ann Surg 1944; 120:417.
18. Avellan L. Reconstruction of defects in the weight bearing surfaces of the foot. Acta Orthop Scand 1965; 36:340–343.
19. London PS. The burned foot. Br J Surg 1953; 40:293–304.
20. Brown JB, McDowell F. Skin grafting of burns. London: Lippincott, 1943.
21. Brou JA, Robson MC, McCauley RL, et al. Inventory of potential reconstructive needs in the patient with burns. J Burn Care Rehabil 1989; 10:555–560.
22. Salisbury RE, Bevin AG. Atlas of Reconstructive Burn Surgery. Philadelphia: WB Saunders, 1981:246–249.
23. Ponsten B. The fasciocutaneous flap; its use in soft tissue defects in the lower limb. Br J Plast Surg 1981; 34:215–220.
24. Tolhurst DE. Clinical experience and complications with fasciocutaneous flaps. Scand J Plast Reconstr Surg 1986; 20:75–78.
25. Tolhurst DE, Haeseker B, Zeeman RJ. The development of the fasciocutaneous flap and its clinical applications. Plast Reconstr Surg 1983; 71:597–606.
26. Barclay TL, Sharp DT, Chisholm EM. Cross-leg fasciocutaneous flaps. Plast Reconstr Surg 1983; 72:843–846.
27. Cormack G, Lamberty BG. A classification of fasciocutaneous flaps according to their pattern of vascularization. Br J Plast Surg 1984; 37;80–87.
28. Maruyama Y, Iwahira Y. Popliteo-posterior thigh fasciocutaneous island flap for closure around the knee. Br J Plast Surg 1989; 42:140–143.
29. Laitung JKG. The lower posterolateral thigh flap. Br J Plast Surg 1989; 42:133–139.
30. McCraw JB, Fishman JH, Sharzer LH. The versatile gastrocnemius myocutaneous flap. Plast Reconstr Surg 1978; 62:15–23.
31. McCraw JB, Dibbell DG, Carraway J. Experimental definition of independent myocutaneous vascular territories. Plast Reconstr Surg 1977; 60:341–352.
32. McCraw JB, Dibbell DG, Carraway J. Clinical definition of independent myocutaneous vascular territories. Plast Reconstr Surg 1977; 60:212–220.

33. Asuku M, McCauley RL. Reconstruction of Burn Deformities of the Lower Extremity. In: McCauley RL, ed. Functional and Aesthetic Reconstruction of Burned Patients. New York: Taylor and Francis, 2005:521–548.
34. Sood R, Ranieri J, Murthy V, et al. The Tibialis Anterior Muscle Flap for Full-Thickness Tibial Burns. J Burn Care Rehabil 2003; 24(6):386–391.
35. Chang J, Most D, Hovey LM, et al. Tibialis anterior turnover flap coverage of the exposed tibia in a severely burned patient. Burns 1997; 23(1):69–71.
36. Hirschowitz B, Moscona R, Kaufman T, et al. External longitudinal splitting of the tibialis anterior muscle for coverage of compound fractures of the middle third of the tibia. Plast Reconstr Surg 1987; 79:407–414.
37. Moller-Larsen F, Petersen NC. Longitudinal split anterior tibial muscle flap with preserved function. Plast Reconstr Surg 1984; 74:398–401.
38. Lo LJ, Chen YR, Weng CJ, Noordhorf MS. Use of split anterior tibial muscle flap in treating avulsion of leg associated with tibial exposure. Ann Plast Surg 1993; 31:112–116.
39. Moscona AR, Govrin-Yehudain J, Hirshowitz B. The island fasciocutaneous flap; a new type of flap for defects of the knee. Br J Plast Surg 1985; 38:512–514.
40. Acland RD, Schusterman M, Godina M, et al. The saphenous neurovascular free flap. Plast Reconstr Surg 1981; 67:763–774.
41. Walton RL, Bunkis J. The posterior calf fasciocutaneous free flap. Plast Reconstr Surg 1984; 74:76–85.
42. Maruyama Y. Bilobed fasciocutaneous flap. Br J Plast Surg 1985; 38:515–517.
43. Heymans O, Verhelle N, Peters S, et al. Use of the medial adipofascial flap of the leg for coverage of full-thickness burns exposing the tibial crest. Burns 2002; 28:674–678.
44. Feller I, Grabb WC. The leg: Principles of treatment. In: Feller I, Grabb WC, eds. Reconstruction and Rehabilitation of the Burned Patient. Dexter, MI: Thomson-Shore Inc., 1979:349–361.
45. Hammer H, Bugyi I, Zellner PR. Soft-tissue reconstruction of the anterior surface of the lower leg in burn patients using a free latissimus dorsi muscle flap. Scand J Plast Reconstr Surg 1986; 20:137–140.
46. Bunkis J, Walton RL, Mathes SJ. The rectus abdominis free flap for lower extremity reconstruction. Ann Plast Surg 1983; 11:373–380.
47. Masquelet MD, Beverage J, Romana C. The lateral supramalleolar flap. Plast Reconstr Surg 1988; 81:74–81.
48. Clark N, Sherman R. Soft-tissue reconstruction of the foot and ankle. Orthop Clin North Am 1993; 24:489–503.
49. Jeng S-F, Wei F-C. Distally based sural island flap for foot reconstruction. Plast Reconstr Surg 1997; 99:744–750.
50. Grabb WC, Argenta LC. The lateral calcaneal artery skin flap. Plast Reconstr Surg 1981; 68:723–730.
51. Rajacic N, Darweesh K, Jayakishnan K, et al. The distally based superficial sural flap for reconstruction of the lower leg and foot. Br J Plast Surg 1996; 49:383–389.
52. Raine TJ, Nahai F. Free tissue transfers to the foot. Plast Surg Forum 1984; 7:112.
53. Hollock GG. The radial forearm flap in burn reconstruction. J Burn Care Rehabil 1986; 7:318–322.
54. Hallock GG. Simultaneous bilateral foot reconstruction using a single free radial forearm flap. Plast Reconstr Surg 1987; 80:836–838.

55. Chicarilli ZN, Ariyan S, Cuono CB. Free radial forearm flap versatility for the head and neck and lower extremity. J Reconstr Microsurg 1986; 2:221–228.
56. Goldberg JA, Adkins P, Tsai T-M. Microvascular reconstruction of the foot: weight bearing patterns, gait analysis, and long-term follow-up. Plast Reconstr Surg 1993; 92:904–911.
57. Uhm K, Shin KS, Lew J. Crane principle of the cross-leg fasciocutaneous flap: aesthetically pleasing technique for damaged dorsum of foot. Ann Plast Surg 1985; 15:257–261.
58. Taylor GA, Hoopson WLG. The cross-foot flap. Plast Reconstr Surg 1975; 55:677–681.
59. Harrison DH, Morgan BDG. The instep island flap to resurface plantar defects. Br J Plast Surg 1981; 34:315–318.
60. Ikuta Y, Murakami T, Yoshioka K, et al. Reconstruction of the heel pad by flexor digitorum brevis musculocutaneous flap transfer. Plast Reconstr Surg 1984; 74:86–96.
61. Gibstein L, Abramson D, Sampson C, et al. Musculofascial flaps based on the dorsalis pedis vascular pedicle for coverage of the foot and ankle. Ann Plast Surg 1996; 37:152–157.
62. Bostwick J. Reconstruction of the heel pad by muscle transposition and split skin graft. Surg Gynaecol Obstet 1976; 143:973–974.
63. Hartrampf CR, Scheflan M, Bostwick J. The flexor digitorum brevis muscle island pedicle flap: a new dimension in heel reconstruction. Plast Reconstr Surg 1980; 66:264–270.
64. Mathes S, Nahai F. Clinical applications for muscle and musculocutaneous flaps. St. Louis CV: Mosby, 1982.
65. Colen LB, Bunke HJ. Neurovascular Island flaps from the plantar vessels and nerves for foot reconstruction. Ann Plast Surg 1984; 12(4):327–332.
66. Landi A, Soragni O, Monteleone M. The extensor digitorum brevis muscle island flap for soft tissue loss around the ankle. Plast Reconstr Surg 1985; 75:892–897.
67. Hong G, Steffenes K, Wang FB. Reconstruction of the lower leg and foot with the reverse pedicle posterior tibial fasciocutaneous flap. Br J Plast Surg 1989; 42:515–516.
68. McCraw JB, Furlow LT. The dorsalis pedis arterialized flap: A clinical study. Plast Reconstr Surg 1975; 55:177–185.
69. Shanahan RE, Gingrass RP. Medial plantar sensory flap for coverage of heel defects. Plast Reconstr Surg 1979; 64:295–298.
70. Morrison WA, Crabb DM, O'Brien BM, et al. The instep of the foot as a fasciocutaneous flap and as a free flap for heel defects. Plast Reconstr Surg 1983; 72:56–63.
71. Stallings JO, Ban JL, Pandeya NK, et al. Secondary burn reconstruction: Recent advances with microvascular free flaps, regional flaps, and specialized grafts. Am Surg 1982; 48:505–513.
72. May JW, Halls MJ, Simon SR. Free microvascular muscle flaps with skin graft reconstruction of extensive defects of the feet: a clinical and gait analysis study. Plast Reconstr Surg 1985; 5:627–641.
73. May JW, Rohrich RJ. Foot reconstruction using free microvascular muscle flaps with skin grafts. Clin Plast Surg 1986; 13:681–689.
74. Maxwell GP, Manson PN, Hoopes JE. Experience with thirteen latissimus dorsi myocutaneous free flaps. Plast Reconstr Surg 1979; 64:1–8.

75. Gordon L, Buncke HJ, Albert BS. Free latissimus dorsi muscle flap with split thickness skin graft cover; a report of sixteen cases. Plast Reconstr Surg 1982; 70:173–178.
76. Bailey BN, Godfrey AM. Latissimus dorsi muscle free flaps. Br J Plast Surg 1982; 35:47–52.
77. Dabb RW, Davis RM. Latissimus dorsi free flap in the elderly: an alternative to below-knee amputation. Plast Reconstr Surg 1984; 73:633–640.
78. Taylor GI, Daniel RK. The free flap: composite tissue transfer by vascular anastomosis. Aust N Z J Surg 1973; 43(1):1–3.
79. Sanger JR, Matloub HS, Gosain AK, et al. Scalp reconstruction with a prefabricated abdominal flap carried by the radial artery. Plast Reconstr Surg 1992; 89(2):315–319.
80. Brenman SA, Barber WB, Pederson WC, et al. Pedicled free flaps: indications in complex reconstruction. Ann Plast Surg 1990; 24:420–426.
81. Mc O'Brien B, Barton RM, Pribaz JJ. The wrist as an immediate free flap carrier for reconstruction of the pelvis: a case report. Br J Plast Surg 1987; 40:427–431.
82. Lai C-S, Lin S-D, Chou C-K, et al. Use of a cross-leg free muscle flap to reconstruct an extensive burn wound involving a lower extremity. Burns 1991; 17(6):510–513.
83. Yamada A, Harii K, Ueda K, et al. Versatility of the cross-leg free rectus abdominis flap for leg reconstruction under difficult and unfavorable conditions. Plast Reconstr Surg 1995; 95(7):1253–1257.
84. Chen HC, Mosely LH, Tang YB, et al. Difficult reconstruction of an extensive injury of the lower extremity with a large cross-leg microvascular composite-tissue flap containing fibula. Plast Reconstr Surg 1989; 83:723–727.
85. Tvrdek M, Pros Z, Nejedly A, et al. Free cross leg flap as a method of reconstruction of soft-tissue defects. Acta Chir Plast 1975; 37(1):12–16.
86. Townsend PL. Indications and long-term assessment of 10 cases of cross-leg free DCIA flaps. Ann Plast Surg 1987; 19(3):225–233.
87. Waymack JP, Fidler J, Warden GD. Surgical correction of burn scar contractures of the foot in children. Burns 1988; 14:156–160.
88. Deitch EA, Wheelaham TM, Paige Rose M, et al. Hypertrophic burn scars: analysis of variables. J Trauma 1983; 23:895–898.
89. Larson DL, Abston S, Willis B, et al. Contracture and scar formation in the burn patient. Clin Plast Surg 1974; 1(4):653–666.
90. Parks DH, Baur PS, Larson DL. Late problems in burns. Clin Plast Surg 1977; 4(4):547–560.
91. Larson DL, Abston S, Evans EB, et al. Techniques of decreasing scar formation and contractures in the burned patient. J Trauma 1971; 11:807–823
92. Perkins K, Davey RB, Wallis KA. Silicon gel: a new treatment for burns scars and contractures. Burns 1982; 9(3):205–213.
93. Bennett GB, Helm P, Purdue GF, et al. Serial casting: a method for treating burn contractures. J Burn Care Rehabil 1989; 10:543–545.
94. Johnson J, Silverberg R. Serial casting of the lower extremity to correct contractures during the acute phase of burn care. Phys Ther 1995; 75:262–266.
95. Achauer BM, Vanderkam VM. Burn reconstruction. In: Achauer BM, ed. Plastic Surgery: Indications, Operations, and Outcomes. Vol.1. St Louis: Mosby, 2000:425–446.

96. Robson MC, Barnett RA, Leitch IO, et al. Prevention and treatment of postburn scar contracture. World J Surg 1992; 16:87–96.
97. Hirshowitz B, Karev A, Mahler D. Proximal and distal releasing incisions for the treatment of flexion contracture of the popliteal region. Br J Plast Surg 1976; 29:35–37.
98. Dhanraj P, Asuku ME, Oh S, McCauley RL. Management of postburn recalcitrant knee ulcers in pediatric patients. J Burn Care Rehabil 2004; 25:129–133.
99. Aarons MS, Lynch JB, Lewis SR. Scar tissue carcinoma: a clinical study with reference to burn scar carcinoma. Ann Surg 1965; 161:170–188.
100. Novick M, Gard DA, Hardy SB, Spira M. Burn scar carcinoma: a review and analysis of 46 cases. J Trauma 1977; 17:809–817.
101. Ozek C, Cankayali R, Ufuk B, et al. Marjolin's ulcers arising in burn scars. J Burn Care and Rehabil 2001; 22(6):384–389.
102. Sarma D, Weilbaecher TG. Carcinoma arising from burn scar. J Surg Onc 1985; 29:89–90.
103. Abbas JS, Beecham JE. Burn wound carcinoma: a case report and review of the literature. Burns 1988; 14(3):222–224.
104. Botswick JPeacock EE, Madden JW, Trier WC. Some studies on the treatment of burned hands. Ann Surg 1970; 171:903.
105. Turley CB, Cutting P, Clarke JA. Medial fasciocutaneous flap of the thigh for release of postburn groin contractures. Br J Plast Surg 1991; 44:36–40.
106. Roberts AHN, Dickson WA. Fasciocutaneous flaps for burn reconstruction: a report of 57 flaps. Br J Plast Surg 1988; 41:150–153.
107. Blackburn JH II, Boemi L, Hall WW, et al. Negative pressure dressings as bolster for skin grafts. Ann Plast Surg 1998; 40(5):453–457.
108. Sposato G, Molea G, Di Caprio G, et al. Ambulant vacuum-assisted closure of skin-graft dressing in the lower limbs using a portable mini-VAC device. Br J Plast Surg 2001; 54(3):235–237.
109. Scherer LA, Shiver S, Chang M, et al. The vacuum assisted closure device: a method of securing skin grafts and improving graft survival. Arch Surg 2002; 137(8):930–934.
110. Webb LX. New techniques in wound management: vacuum-assisted wound closure. J Am Acad Orthop Surg 2002; 10(5):303–311.
111. Wang TN, Whetzel T, Mathes SJ, et al. A fasciocutaneous flap for vaginal and perineal reconstruction. Plast Reconstr Surg 1987; 80:95–103.
112. Hayashi A, Maruyama Y. The use of the anteromedial thigh fasciocutaneous flap in the reconstruction of the lower abdomen and inguinal region; a report of two cases. Br J Plast Surg 1988; 41:633–638.
113. Song YG, Chen GZ, Song YL. The free thigh flap: a new free flap concept based on the septo cutaneous artery. Br J Plast Surg 1984; 37:149–159.
114. Bostwick J, Hill HL, Nahai F. Repairs in the lower abdomen, groin, or perineum with myocutaneous or omental flaps. Plast Reconstr Surg 1979; 63:186–194.
115. Gopinath KS, Chandrashekhar M, Kumar MV, Srikant KC. Tensor fasciae latae myocutaneous flaps to reconstruct skin defects after radical inguinal lymphadenectomy. Br J Plast Surg 1988; 41:366–368.
116. Prakash V. A new concept for the management of postburn contractures. Plast Reconstr Surg 2000; 106(1):233–234.
117. Prakash V, Bajaj SP. Flap stretching for management of postburn knee contracture with unstable scar. Plast Reconstr Surg 2001; 108(2):587–588.

118. Prakash V, Mishra A. Use of posterior calf fascial flap: a new concept for the management of knee contracture with unstable scar. Plast Reconstr Surg 2003; 111(1):505.
119. Robert L, Walton W, Matory E, et al. The posterior calf fascial free flap. Plast Reconstr Surg 1985; 76:914–924.
120. Ahmad CN, Ashraf DM. Z-lengthening and gastrocnemius muscle flap in the management of severe postburn flexion contractures of the knee. Journal of Trauma 1998; 45(1):127–132.
121. Abraham E, Verinder DGR, Sharrard WJW. The treatment of flexion contracture of the knee in myelomeningocele. J Bone Joint Surg Br 1977; 59:433–438.
122. Aydan A. An unusual contracture of the foot caused by a neglected burn wound salvaged by a cross-leg flap. Plast Reconstr Surg 2002; 110(5):1373.
123. Rose EH, Norris MS. The versatile temporoparietal fascial flap: adaptability to a variety of composite defects. Plast Reconstr Surg 1990; 85(2):224–232.
124. Fernandez-Palacios J, DeArmas DF, Deniz HV, et al. Radial free flaps in plantar burns. Burns 1996; 22:242–245.
125. Ramakrishnan KM, Ch M, Jayaramoan V, et al. Deepithelialized turnover flaps in burns. Plast Reconstr Surg 1988; 82:262–266.
126. Pap AS. Hot metal burns of the feet in foundry workers. J Occup Med 1966; 8:537.
127. Dhanraj P, Faro O, Phillips LG, McCauley RL. Burn scar contractures of the feet: efficacy of bilateral simultaneous surgical correction. Burns 2002; 28(8):814–819.

9

Wound Healing and Tissue Engineering

Physiology of Wound Healing

Zubin J. Panthaki

Departments of Clinical Surgery, Clinical Orthopedics, and Rehabilitation, Division of Plastic and Hand Surgery, DeWitt Daughtry Family Department of Surgery, Miller School of Medicine, University of Miami, Miami, Florida, U.S.A.

Anire Okpaku

Department of Surgery, Jackson Memorial Hospital, Miller School of Medicine, University of Miami, Miami, Florida, U.S.A.

INTRODUCTION

In order to understand the pathophysiology of the traumatized lower extremity, one must first understand the classical phases of wound healing:

1. inflammatory (lag) phase,
2. repair (proliferative) phase, and
3. maturation (remodeling) phase.

Inflammatory (Lag) Phase

The inflammatory phase of wound healing is initiated by injury: be it trauma, infection, or antigen–antibody reaction; and is nonspecific in response. The body's immediate response to injury is multifaceted and nonspecific.

The response begins with vasoconstriction and is the body's attempt to achieve hemostasis and formation of a fibrin clot. It lasts about 5 to 10 minutes.

Platelet aggregates form as a result of exposed subendothelial collagen and this is then followed by platelet degranulation, which releases multiple growth factors into the immediate wound environment. The intrinsic and extrinsic coagulation cascades are also initiated.

Next comes a vasodilatory phase where blood flow to the wound environment increases tenfold. Gaps form between endothelial cells in the local wound. Leukocytes marginate and then migrate through these gaps and release a variety of vasoactive substances. These include amines (histamines and serotonin), polypeptides (bradykinin), and eicosanoids (prostaglandins).

The vasodilatory phase leads to the recruitment of inflammatory cells to the wound site. These cells initially adhere to the damaged endothelium through the action of selectins, and then in a more forceful way through beta-2 integrins. The circulating monocytes that become fixed in tissue in this fashion are macrophages. They act as the control cells of wound repair, secreting almost all growth factors and cytokines and regulating matrix production and degradation, angiogenesis, and epithelialization. Polymorphonuclear leukocytes are also recruited to the wound site, and they play a short-lived role for control of infection but are not directly needed for wound healing.

Repair (Proliferative) Phase

Because inflammation subsides, wound repair commences. This is the second phase, also known as the proliferative or fibroplasia phase of wound healing. This process can start as early as the third day after injury. Epidermal cells from the edge of the wound begin to migrate forward to cover the surface of the wound (1). At the same time, fibroblasts from the perivascular tissue migrate into the wound along the fibrin matrix and secrete glycosaminoglycans, fibronectin, and collagen matrices. Type III collagen is initially formed before type I. Because the proliferative phase progresses, wound tensile strength increases proportionately to the collagen content for the first three weeks. Then, although wound strength continues to increase, the net collagen production slows down because synthesis and degradation come into equilibrium around six weeks postinjury.

Maturation (Remodeling) Phase

The remodeling phase occurs after closure of the wound has taken place. The remodeling occurs over months to years and involves a decrease in cellular contents and blood flow (2). The wound continues to gain strength during the maturation phase despite no net increase in collagen. This comes about through three mechanisms:

1. Collagen that was initially laid down in a haphazard manner gets reoriented along mechanical stress lines.
2. More stable bonds are formed within the proteoglycans and collagen molecules.
3. The embryonic type III collagen that was laid down early gets replaced with normal, mature, type I collagen.

Because the wound continues to mature, it approaches the collagen ratio of types I to III collagen of 4:1 of normal adult skin.

The extent to which each component/process plays a role in the wound healing process depends also on the type of injury. Superficial skin wounds, such as abrasions, split-thickness skin graft donor sites, or partial thickness burns, as well as venous stasis ulcers, heal almost entirely by epithelialization. Deep chronic pressure ulcers require extensive matrix synthesis, angiogenesis, fibroplasia, and contraction. Diabetic foot ulcers require angiogenesis, deposition of extracellular matrix, contraction, and epithelialization (3).

FACTORS THAT AFFECT THE WOUND HEALING ENVIRONMENT

In addition to the direct limb damage from high-energy trauma, traumatic injuries involving burns, cold injury, pressure injury, and radiation may result in the development of wounds.

Intrinsic Factors

A variety of factors impact wound healing. These factors are listed in Table 1. Some factors are more significant than others. In fact, it is estimated that 45% to 70% of all lower extremity amputations are in patients with diabetes (4). Furthermore, the aging process results in a variety of histological changes to the skin that can impact wound healing (Table 2) (5).

Traditional Wound Care

The debridement of necrotic tissue by either surgical or nonsurgical means is an essential component of wound care. Failure to adequately debride necrotic tissue in a timely manner leads to a delay in wound healing and can potentially lead to wound infection.

While the effectiveness of occlusive dressings in improving healing rates is difficult to demonstrate clinically, they often decrease pain and improve convenience of use and cost-effectiveness (2). Only dressings containing hyaluronic acid have been shown to specifically promote healing (2).

Table 1 Comorbidities Associated with Poor Wound Healing

Vascular (arteriosclerosis, vasculitis, lymphedema, venous stasis)
Neuropathic (diabetes)
Hematologic (dysproteinemia, red blood cell disorders)
Neoplasms
Infections (bacterial and fungal)

Source: From Ref. 4.

Table 2 Skin Changes with Aging

Epidermis
Flattened dermal–epidermal junction
Decreased epidermal turnover rate
Slower formation of neutral lipids in the stratum corneum
Fewer melanocytes
Fewer Langerhans cells
Dermis
Atrophy
Fewer fibroblasts
Fewer mast cells
Fewer blood vessels
Increased blood vessel variability in size
Shortened capillary loops
Abnormal nerve endings

Even with these measures, many patients fail to heal their wounds. For example, the nonoperative treatment of pressure ulcers shows long-term healing rates of 39.9% for stage III and 34.1% for stage IV in nursing home patients and 45.2% and 30.6% for hospitalized patients (6). Operative therapy can consist of debridement, primary closure, or skin grafts. For more severe injuries, myocutaneous or fasciocutaneous flaps may be needed. Hallock (7) noted that one-third of all patients receiving a muscle or fascial flap for a lower extremity traumatic injury had a postoperative complication. In addition, operative therapy with flaps is only successful in 31% of patients with pressure ulcers (6).

Given these poor long-term healing rates, there has been much basic and clinical research devoted to new treatments for lower extremity wounds. The following sections highlight some of the new treatments. It is important to remember that many patients require a multimodality approach to the treatment of their injuries.

Extrinsic (Modifiable) Factors

Systemic Therapies

Pentoxifylline (800 mg three times a day) may be a helpful adjunct in the healing of lower extremity wounds (8). As an inhibitor of tumor necrosis factor-α, pentoxifylline acts to reduce leukocyte adhesion and improve red blood cell flow through the microvasculature (9). Unfortunately, the clinical data have not shown this agent to be effective in increasing healing rates of leg wounds (9). The anabolic steroid stanozolol may be effective in treating ulcers due to lipodermatosclerosis and cryofibrinogenemia, but has no effect on other types of leg wounds (4).

Hyperbaric Oxygen Therapy

Adequate tissue oxygenation is necessary for all phases of wound healing. The ability of leukocytes to kill bacteria is impeded by low partial pressure of oxygen. Angiogenesis, collagen synthesis, and epithelialization are also inhibited. A periwound oxygen pressure of 30 mmHg may suggest that there is insufficient oxygen at the injury site for effective healing (3). Tissue hypoxia can often be treated with surgical revascularization and by addressing anemia, hypovolemia, hypoxia, and vasospasm. Hyperbaric oxygen therapy has been suggested as a useful adjunct in the care of patients with difficult-to-heal wounds from the following types of injuries:

- acute crush injuries,
- prior radiation therapy,
- aggressive soft-tissue infections,
- nonhealing ulcers, and
- compromised skin grafts and flaps.

With regard to lower extremity wounds, the data regarding the effectiveness of hyperbaric oxygen therapy are scarce, involving only small numbers of patients and often difficult to interpret (10). In addition, there are contraindications and side effects of hyperbaric oxygen therapy.

Contraindications to Hyperbaric Oxygen Therapy (11)

- Absolute
  untreated pneumothorax
- Relative
  obstructive lung disease,
  upper respiratory or sinus infections,
  recent ear surgery or injury,
  fever,
  claustrophobia.

Side Effects of Hyperbaric Oxygen Therapy (11)

- reversible myopia (occurs in up to 20% of patients),
- symptomatic otic barotrauma (occurs in up to 3–20% of patients),
- pulmonary oxygen toxicity, and
- seizures (rare).

Topical Growth Factors

The normal function of growth factors is to attract various cell types into the wound, stimulate cellular proliferation, stimulate epithelialization, promote angiogenesis, and regulate synthesis and degradation of extracellular matrix. It has been hypothesized that pressure ulcers, and possibly other chronic wounds, may be deficient in one or more growth factors (6). While standard occlusive dressings may provide an appropriate environment for wound healing, growth factors may still be deficient in this microenvironment. Clinical results from topical application of growth factors to chronic wounds have not been as dramatic

Table 3 Contraindications to the Use of Regranex (Becaplermin) Gel

Known hypersensitivity to any component of the gel
Known neoplasm at the site of application
Uncontrolled wound infection
Wounds with ankle-brachial index of <0.45 or transcutaneous pressure of oxygen <30 mmHg at the ankle
Wounds exposed to repetitive trauma
Grossly draining wounds
Patients receiving chemotherapy, radiation therapy, or steroids (>15 mg prednisone/day)

as first hoped. This is unsurprising when one considers the complexity of the wound healing process.

Topical growth factors have been shown to improve the long-term outcomes of patients with diabetic ulcers and pressure ulcers (6,12). To date, only platelet-derived growth factor has been licensed for use, for treating noninfected foot ulcers up to 5 cm^2 in diabetic patients (becaplermin, Regranex). Endogenous platelet-derived growth factors are produced by platelets, monocytes, macrophages, endothelial cells, fibroblasts, or smooth muscle cells (13). Research studies have shown that it may also have some value in lower extremity wounds due to pressure, venous, iatrogenic, and post-surgical etiology (13,14). Table 3 lists the contraindications to the use of Regranex gel (13).

Although not yet licensed, granulocyte colony-stimulating factor has been evaluated for treating infected foot ulcers in diabetic patients and was associated with more rapid resolution of cellulitis and decreased antibiotic requirements. Furthermore, fibroblast growth factor has been assessed for treating pressure ulcers. Epidermal growth factor and transforming growth factor B are currently being studied for the treatment of venous ulcers (2).

In the future, growth factors may be administered sequentially, in combination, or at timed intervals to more closely mimic the normal healing process. The diversity of growth factors and types of chronic wound suggest that these factors have potential as new treatments if patients' individual requirements can be identified.

TISSUE ENGINEERING

Classically, tissue bioengineering implies the use of organ-specific cells that seed a scaffold ex vivo. Postnatal stem cells are often needed in order to regenerate sustainable tissue, such as skin and bone. The isolation of these "self-renewing" stem cells also offers an opportunity for future gene therapy interventions (15). We will briefly discuss the current status of tissue engineering in various tissue types.

Cartilage

Cartilage is a complex tissue consisting of cartilage matrix (composed of collagens and proteoglycan aggregates). The repair of cartilage caused by trauma may require either an allogenic cartilage transplant or the implantation of autologous chondrocytes (16). For younger patients (less than 50 years of age) osteochondral shell allografts and autographs have been shown to be effective in resurfacing the knee (16). Stem cells cultured with transforming growth factor-beta one (TGFB1) offer another strategy for autologous chondrocytes. Mesenchymal stem cells (MSCs) are important potential sites for obtaining these cells. MSCs are found in the bone marrow in low numbers and are capable of differentiating into chondrocytes, osteocytes, myocytes, and adipocytes. They can be amplified rapidly in culture 2000-fold in about 10 days (16). This strategy may be helpful for older patients who have underlying chronic cartilage inflammation (16).

Bone

Table 4 lists the traditional treatments for large segmental osseous defects and their clinical limitations (17).

Tissue bioengineering is more difficult for bone (which requires a three-dimensional construct as well as an internal architecture) than skin, which forms essentially a two-dimensional sheet. Tissue engineering techniques have been used in a variety of settings to produce new cartilage from autologous isolated chondrocytes (18). Engineering new cartilage is more difficult than bone. Cartilage is nearly avascular and is devoid of progenitor cells.

Bone morphogenetic proteins (BMPs) are members of the transforming growth factor-beta (TGF-B) superfamily of proteins, (19) which stimulate MSCs to differentiate into chondroblasts and osteoblasts. BMPs also have chemostatic properties that draw osteoblasts to the site of bone growth as well as osteoinduction properties that differentiate osteoblasts and chondroblasts into mature, terminally differentiated cells. BMPs may have the potential to stimulate bone growth

Table 4 Treatment Options for Large Segmental Osseous Defects and Their Clinical Limitations

Autogenous bone grafts	Limited by donor site availability Donor site morbidity
Allogenic grafting	Risk of infection Major histoincompatibility Graft vs. host disease Need for immunosuppression
Nondegradable materials	
Metals	Stress shielding (leading to deterioration of surrounding bone)
Ceramics	Structural failure
Cements	High rate of infection

where gaps exist due to trauma, osteomyelitis, cancer, or other injuries (19). BMPs may also be helpful to stabilize implant services and titanium screws (19).

Johnson et al. (20) studied the use of an autolysed antigen-free cortical allograft lyophilized with human BMP in 30 patients who had failure of femoral fracture healing. Twenty-eight of 30 patients healed with this technique (21), compared with the use of the BMP, osteogenic protein-1 in a type 1 collagen carrier to bone autographs in 124 patients with tibial nonunions (21). Healing rates and complications were similar in the two groups except that 20% of patients treated with autographs had chronic pain at the donor site.

Skeletal stem cells (bone-marrow stromal stem cells) are able to undergo extensive replication in culture and can form bone, cartilage, and adipocytes in vivo (15). These stem cells must be combined with appropriate scaffolding before they can be used in vivo. A variety of biocompatible polymeric scaffolds are being developed to address the limitations listed in Table 2. These scaffolds will have the following advantages:

- minimal loss of cells from the target area,
- one-way communication allows growth factors to diffuse outward while preventing immunological cells such as T-cells and macrophages from entering the site.

An important limitation to these bioengineered scaffolds is the limited mechanical support. While the first clinical trials using skeletal stem cells cultures loaded on an appropriate carrier will be used to repair large size bone defects, genetically altered stem cells may be used in the future to treat a variety of crippling genetic diseases.

Skin

Split thickness skin grafts often result in pain, infection, and donor site morbidity. The use of cadaveric allografts is complicated by immunorejection (17). The use of epidermal autographs (where small amounts of skin are cultured to produce large amounts of epidermal sheets) has fallen out of favor because this procedure is technically difficult and has had only limited clinical success (2). However, the potential benefits of skin engineering led to the development of skin equivalents, in which donor tissue with limited immunogenicity is used. There are now several commercially available products.

Commercially Available Skin Substitutes

Another alternative is the use of alloderm, which is a cadaveric graft that has been treated chemically to remove cells, leaving just the acellular dermal matrix and intact basement membrane complex. Because it is immunologically inert, this product may have a role in the treatment of deep-partial and full-thickness wounds (17).

Graftskin (Apligraf) is a bilayered skin construct that has been approved for use in the healing of lower extremity venous ulcers and diabetic foot ulcers. Although the exact mechanism is unclear, it is believed that the graft acts as a matrix that recruits cells to the wound bed. Graftskin incorporates cultured allogeneic keratinocytes and fibroblasts from neonatal foreskin on a bovine type I collagen dermal matrix. Apligraf has been shown to accelerate the rate of wound healing and to be cost-effective (8). Integra is a combination of dermal fibroblasts and bovine collagen.

Dermagraft consists of nonimmunogenic neonatal fibroblast cultured on a polyglactin mesh and has been shown to lead to more complete and rapid healing of diabetic foot ulcers compared with conventional therapy. Although the mechanism by which this dermal tissue promotes wound healing is unknown, it is believed that it is a result of the matrix components and cytokines produced by the cultured fibroblasts (22). All these products have been used to treat burns.

Integra bilayer wound matrix (Integra Lifesciences Corporation) is a synthetic skin substitute comprised of a porous matrix of cross-linked bovine tendon collagen and glycosaminoglycan and a semi-permeable polysiloxane (silicone) layer. The semi-permeable silicone membrane controls water vapor loss, provides a flexible adherent covering for the wound surface and adds increased tear strength to the device. The collagen-glycosaminoglycan biodegradable matrix provides a scaffold for cellular invasion and capillary growth.

Fibrin Glue

Fibrin glue has been used as an adhesive with skin grafts and tissue-engineered skin substitutes. A variety of commercial products are available. Most of these products consist of cryoprecipitated fibrinogen and fibronectin, thrombin, calcium chloride, and factor XIII (23). Studies have shown that fibrin glue can reduce hemorrhage associated with skin grafting. Fibrin glue may also improve graft adherence and take. By stabilizing the graft and promoting graft nutrition and angiogenesis, the fibrin glue helps keep the skin graft site sterile. Fibrin glue also has the potential to serve as a template for cellular migration, a delivery system for cultured keratinocytes and fibroblasts, and as a delivery system for growth factors (23).

Nerve

The most common injury involving peripheral nerves is a sharp cut that severs the nerve cable. In such cases, the proximal portion of the nerve remains viable while the distal segment atrophies. The nerve cables surrounding the distal nerve segment often remain intact and may serve as a potential channel for the proximal axon to regenerate (24,25). The results of peripheral neurorrhaphy under tension have been disappointing, especially if the distance between the two ends is greater than 1 cm (26,27). In such cases, a nerve graft may be used. This procedure involves harvesting a section of another nerve, usually the sural nerve, which is then used to fill the gap at the site of injury. In lower extremity injuries, this may not be an available option.

The use of nerve allografts has not been effective due to the host immune response (24). In order to avoid the donor morbidity associated with autologous nerve grafts, other autologous tissue grafts are an alternative. Muscle and vein tubes can be used as a scaffolding template graft to reconnect the injured nerve. The recovery of function may not be as good as with nerve grafts. Work is in progress, however, to improve the success of such matrices by implantation of cultured Schwann cells (28).

A variety of other techniques to develop nerve conduits are currently under development. One involves the development of a conduit channel wall. This wall can be made from natural materials (vein, laminin, fibronectin, and collagen), nonbiodegradable synthetic materials (silicone), and biodegradable synthetic materials [(polylactic acid/ polyglycolic acid, polyurethane, poly (organo) phosphazenes)] (24).

REFERENCES

1. Martin P. Wound healing-aiming for perfect skin regeneration. Science 1997; 276:75–81.
2. Harding KG, Morris HL, Patel GK. Healing chronic wounds. Br Med J 2002; 324:160–163.
3. Robson MC, Mustoe TA, Hunt TK. The future of recombinant growth factors in wound healing. Am J Surg 1998; 176:80S–82S.
4. Resnick HE, Valsania P, Phillips CL. Diabetes mellitus and nontraumatic lower extremity amputation in black and white Americans: the National Health and Nutrition Examination Survey Epidemiologic Follow-up study, 1971–1992. Arch Intern Med 1999; 159(20):2470–2475.
5. Yaar Mina, Gilchrest BA. Skin aging. Clin Geriatr Med 2001; 17:617.
6. Payne WG, Ochs DE, Meltzer DD, et al. Long-term outcome study of growth factor-treated pressure ulcers. Am J Surg 2001; 181:81–86.
7. Hallock GG. Utility of both muscle and fascia flaps in severe lower extremity trauma. J Trauma 2000; 48:913–917.
8. Paquette D, Falanga V. Leg ulcers. Clin Geriatr Med 2002; 18:77–88.
9. Dale JJ, Ruckley CV, Harper DR, Gibson B, Nelson EA, Prescott RJ. Randomised, double blind placebo controlled trial of pentoxifylline in the treatment of venous leg ulcers. Br Med J 1999; 319:875–878.
10. Ciaravino ME, Friedell ML, Kammerlocher TC. Is hyperbaric oxygen a useful adjunct in the management of problem lower extremity wounds? Ann Vasc Surg 1996; 10:558–562.
11. Leach RM, Rees PJ, Wilmshurst P. ABC of oxygen: hyperbaric oxygen therapy. Br Med J 1998; 317:1140–1143.
12. Steed DL, Donohoe D, Webster MW, Lindsley L. Effect of extensive debridement and treatment on the healing of diabetic foot ulcers. Diabetic Ulcer Study Group. J Am Coll Surg 1996; 183(1):61–64.

13. Mulder GD. Standardizing wound treatment procedures for advanced technologies. J Am Podiatr Med Assoc 2002; 92:7–11.
14. Kallianinen LK, Hirshberg J, Marchant B, Rees RS. Role of platelet-dervied growth factor as an adjunct to surgery in the management of pressure ulcers. Plast Resconstr Surg 2000; 106:1243–1248.
15. Bianco P, Robey PG. Stem cells in tissue engineering. Nature 2001; 414:118–121.
16. Jorgensen C, Noel D, Apparailly F, Sany J. Stem cells for repair of cartilage and bone: the next challenge in osteoarthritis and rheumatoid arthritis. Ann Rheum Dis 2001; 60:305–309.
17. Warren SM, Longaker MT. New directions in plastic surgery research. Clin Plast Surg 2001; 28:719–730.
18. Nasseri BA, Ogawa K, Vacanti JP. Tissue engineering: an evolving 21st century science to provide biologic replacement for reconstruction and transplantation. Surgery 2001; 130:781–782.
19. Cheng SL, Lou J, Wright NM, Lai CF, Avioli LV, Riew KD. In vitro and in vivo induction of bone formation using a recombinant adenoviral vector carrying the human BMP-2 gene. Calcif Tissue Int 2001; 68(2):87–94.
20. Johnson CS, Preuss HS, Eriksson E. Plastic surgery. In: Courtney M. Townsend Jr., ed. Sabiston Textbook of Surgery: The Biological Basis of Modern Surgical Practice. 16th ed. Philadelphia: WB Saunders Co., 2001:1550–1569.
21. Friedlaender GE, Perry CR, Cole JD, et al. Osteogenic protein-1 (bone morphogenetic protein-7) in the treatment of tibial nonunions. J Bone Joint Surg Am 2001; 83-A Suppl 1(Pt 2):S151–158.
22. Gentzkow GD, Iwasaki SD, Hershon KS, et al. Use of dermagraft, a cultured human dermis, to treat diabetic foot ulcers. Diab Care 1996; 19:350–354.
23. Currie DJ, Sharpe JR, Martin R. The use of fibrin glue in skin grafts and tissue-engineered skin replacements: a review. Plast Reconstr Surg 2001; 108:1713–1726.
24. Hudson TW, Evans GR, Schmidt CE. Engineering strategies for peripheral nerve repair. Orthop Clin North Am 2000; 31:485–498.
25. Brushart T. New strategies for nerve regeneration. Available at www.hopkinsmedicine.org/orthopedicsurgery/news/ws1997/under.html (accessed March 27, 2002).
26. Millesi H. Nerve grafting. Clin Plast Surg 1984; 11:105–113.
27. Brushart TM, Hoffman PN, Royall RM, Murinson BB, Witzel C, Gordon T. Electrical stimulation promotes motoneuron regeneration without increasing its speed or conditioning the neuron. J Neurosci 2002; 22(15):6631–6638.
28. Fansa H, Schneider W, Wolf G, Keilhoff G. Host responses after a cellular muscle basal lamina allografting used as a matrix for tissue engineered nerve grafts. Transplantation 2002; 74:381–387.

Index